As a book editor, I encoun[...] genres, and writing styles. Warren Selkow's book resonates like no other.

The impact of Warren's presentation exceeds anything a medical professional could achieve in educating at-risk people about the immediate need for lifestyle changes. With its perceptive commentary from coauthor Donna Selkow, this book is a must-read for patients and caregivers. Physicians who treat patients with chronic disease, regardless of etiology, will benefit too.

The Simplified Handbook for Living with Heart Disease may even be a lifesaver.

Gail Chadwick, Editor

"I have found the book very interesting and I think everyone over forty years of age should read it. This book explains the pain before the heart attack, the pain while having the attack, and your recovery from it all. When you are at home with the family, you all have concerns at that time, and the book explains how to appreciate these concerns for the betterment of all."

Paul Beck
Cardiac Patient

"Mr. Selkow has written a no-holds-barred, front-row account that every heart patient should read.
It is thought provoking, amusing, hard hitting and direct.
I will give it to all my cardiac patients."

Dr. Edward Kowaleski,
Internal Medicine, Medical Director, Banner Arizona
Medical Clinic, Peoria, Arizona.

"WOW! This fast reading handbook has invaluable facts and tips for the heart patient to be, the recovering patient, and the caregiver. It convinced this patient to follow prescribed diet and medicines.

Jim Sterling, Glendale Arizona
Cardiac Patient

The Simplified Handbook for Living with Heart Disease is an excellent personal insight into the process of learning to live with heart disease and tools to change your lifestyle to live to your life's full expectancy."

Mark Bank, MS, CES, Manager, Banner Boswell Center Cardiac Rehabilitation Program

I feel the chapter on depression and stress is a very honest documentation of how this disease affected Warren. It can affect every person differently. The important fact to remember is that depression and stress are sometimes unavoidable and must be acknowledged and treated for the healing process to begin.

Leanne Kedzie, RN, CLNC, Banner Boswell Hospital, Peoria, Arizona

"Well done, easy to follow for the layperson. Congrats."
Dr. Darry Johnson, Neurologist, Peoria, Arizona

"Warren shares a wealth of hard-won experience to help others understand what they are going through. As a caregiver, I especially appreciated the additional perspective of living through the trials and at times frustrations that loved ones go through when caring for a heart surgery patient. I recommend this book to those who will be going through a heart surgery, have just had heart surgery, or who are trying to figure out what their new lifestyle must be to survive for years to come. I also, and maybe more so, recommend this book to the people who, out of love, will care for a husband, wife, parent, or sibling. The advice is down to earth and realistic—it will help."

Dan Morris, Caregiver, Downers Grove, Illinois. Dan wanted to be listed this way; he is a friend who is traveling the same path as every family caregiver group.

"Warren cuts to the essential issues in a no-nonsense manner which I approve."

John S. Wohleen, BMinE (Ret), Arizona

"The Simplified Handbook for Living with Heart Disease is an outstanding, educational resource with an emphasis on health promotion for anyone with, or at risk for, coronary artery disease. This book is written by the patient and his caregiver who speak from their experiences, with a humorous but serious, insightful, easy-to-read style."

Ellen Webb, RN, BSN, CNOR, Tucson, Arizona

I can open *The Simplified Handbook for Living with Heart Disease* to any page and my attention is immediately grabbed by the message on that page, and all that follows. Fear had a tight hold of me when I learned my loved one needed a bypass. I knew I needed an understanding of what we were facing, but had no idea how to achieve that insight, until I received this remarkable book. I remain fearful, but at least I know why and what to do about it.

Lorraine M. Bell, Caregiver and RN, Sun City, Arizona

Engaging, sarcastic (but honest), AND educational…who knew? Live long and prosper.

Krishna S Schiller, PharmD, Clinical Pharmacist, Banner Good Samaritan Hospital, Phoenix, Arizona

Having had a heart attack nearly ten years ago, I truly enjoyed this book! It would be a welcome reading on what to expect following heart problems. So much is unfamiliar to the new "zipper world."

Betty Budler, Sun City, Arizona

This is a potentially life-changing book applicable to millions. It is a very informative and accurate medical book written from a unique perspective, the patient. Warren combines the personal experience of enduring a serious health problem with the ability to understands complex medical principles and effectively communicate it in a manner all can understand. Additionally, his message is provided with the persuasive vigor only a successful businessman can deliver. It is powerful message that clearly stands to favorably affect the lives of those that desire to prevent heart disease or reduce the likelihood of its progression. Also, for anyone entering the healthcare system for diagnostic or therapeutic cardiac services they will receive an accurate account of what to expect and how to avoid pitfalls.

Additionally, as a cardiologist who has made a career in trying to communicate complex principles to motivate successful lifesaving changes, I have learned a great deal in reading this book. The insights provided by Warren's experience will empower me to deliver a more effective message to my patients.

Dr. T. Gregory Quinn, Cardiologist, board certified cardiology with Sutter East Bay Medical Foundation, Oakland, California, specializing in interventional medicine.

The Simplified Handbook for Living with Heart Disease is based upon Warren Selkow's personal experience as a patient who had open heart surgery and his wife Donna who cared for him during this challenging time and afterwards. This wonderful book about their journey together provides the valuable insight and information for every person with heart disease. May it serve as a guide for those who are overwhelmed, fearful or confused so they may truly understand what is at stake and how to not only live with heart disease but improve their health as well.

Dr. Mark Nelson, Cardiologist, Board Certified in Cardiology and Internal Medicine, Troy, New York

As you'll soon see, Mr. Selkow is a "no frills" kind of guy. He gives it to you straight and pulls no punches on himself or the medical system as it pertains to recovery from heart disease.

Michael Cofield, PhD, ABPP Clinical Health Psychologist, Peoria, Arizona

If you have a victim mentality or are faint of heart- move on! Otherwise, read and learn an important lesson about taking charge of your health and living your life to the fullest.

Mary Ann Zimmerman, MC, LPC Managing Director, Ultra Learning Systems, LLC and the Mindability Group

Warren Selkow's The Simplified Handbook for Living with Heart Disease is a book written by a patient for a patient. This hard-hitting personal story is not a medical book, though Warren covers the basics well. It is a book about what it really means from a patient's perspective to suffer and survive a massive heart attack and live with severe chronic heart disease. This book is brutally honest, an engaging read and, most importantly, the kick in the pants that some people may need to recapture their health.

Mark Moeller, MD, Family Practice Physician, Co-founder of MedHealth Solutions, a web-based company offering health behavioral change solutions for disease prevention and health optimization. Davis, CA.

The Simplified Handbook for Living with Heart Disease

AND OTHER CHRONIC DISEASES

Warren Selkow, PATIENT
Donna Selkow, CAREGIVER

Forward by Dr. Joseph Caplan, Cardiologist

ISBN: 1-4392-4546-0
ISBN-13: 9781439245460
Library of Congress Control Number: 2009905863

Visit www.booksurge.com to order additional copies.

Table of Contents

A Fable[1]

A carter[2] was hauling a load of firewood to a nearby town after a heavy rainfall. The road was muddy. His cart became mired in the mud. No matter how hard he beat his ass, the poor animal could not pull the cart free. The carter cried to his favorite god Hercules for help. If you have some heavy lifting to do, Hercules is the go-to god.

Hercules showed up and asked, "What is the problem?" (Have you ever noticed in fables that gods ask some really dumb questions?) The carter pointed to his mired wheel and asked for help.

Hercules looked the situation over and said to the carter, "Get off your cart and pull on the ass's harness." The carter complied but no matter how hard he pulled and no matter how hard the ass pulled, the cart would not budge.

When Hercules saw they were not making progress, he said, "Take half the load off the cart." The carter complied and, once again, he and his ass pulled and pulled but still to no avail.

Hercules then said, "Take the rest of the load off the cart." The carter once again complied but this time, when he and the ass pulled, the cart immediately broke free of the mud. The carter reloaded his cart and, giving great thanks to Hercules, resumed his trip.

Moral: The gods help those that help themselves.

෧

---

1   Fables are attributed to Aesop (620–560 BC), a slave and storyteller who lived in ancient Greece.

2   Carter is an ancient term used to describe what today would be called a trucker.

Foreword

About two years ago, I accepted a new cardiac patient. Normally this is nothing unique or exceptional. I have a practice with offices in Peoria and Sun City, Arizona. All of the patients I see are suffering from some form of coronary artery disease (CAD) or congestive heart failure (CHF). My patients, like most cardiologists' patients, exhibit a wide range of attitudes as regards how well they comply (or don't comply) with the directions they receive. There is nothing special about my practice in this respect.

This new patient, Warren Selkow, was different from any I had ever seen. He wanted to know everything. He literally challenged me to explain why one course of action was different from another prescribed regimen and, more importantly, what he could expect. He also, reluctantly, agreed to enter the Wellness Clinics that are part of my practice. These clinics provide both a patient education experience and a unique clinical approach to chronic disease management. After our first few visits, I started to get a different "vibe" from this man.

It turned out he had good reason for being so demanding. He had survived two very serious open-heart surgeries and he was still in the process of getting his life together, this several years after the last surgery. He had made the mental leap that survival was not easy and one of the key factors for success was a complete understanding of the underlying problems.

One day, unsolicited and unexpectedly, I received a monograph from Mr. Selkow entitled, "Confessions of a Foodaholic." In about fifteen pages, my patient had created the start of a "core" curriculum, not for doctors, but for patients. Not only that, the insights and advice given in this short piece applied not to heart patients, but to sufferers of many chronic diseases including renal failure, pulmonary disease, and diabetes. This was important, as many heart patients suffer from more than one illness.

In our first visit after I received this monograph, I asked him why he had written the work. His answer was alarmingly simple. "If I had only known all that stuff at the outset of my illness I would have avoided much aggravation and grief. Nobody tells you. You are unprepared. You live a hard life thinking you are alone and nobody else has suffered the same things. I think this paper could help others understand, prepare them, and make life a little easier."

I asked him if he could expand and expound on the work. He went away grumbling about not wanting to get too involved, as he was too lazy to do much work. It seems I had unleashed a tiger. All I had wanted was a more complete piece that I could use in my practice as part of my Wellness Clinics. That is not what he came up with. He kind of exceeded my expectations.

What he wrote is a definitive book on literally everything a heart disease patient needs to know. To accomplish what is essentially a complete treatise on the subject, he wrote about eight years of experiences with the disease, starting with his very first heart attack. Moreover, he applied his considerable skill to analyze and detail what he did wrong to facilitate that first heart attack and what the impacts of the mistakes were. Mostly, he pointed out where the real accountability lies for the disease.

Now it would be possible to believe the book is a sob story about one man's journey. That would be incorrect. Instead, my patient turned a steady and calm hand to the problem and wrote about it in an entertaining, concise—to the point of being blunt in some cases—and informative manner. If this were all he accomplished, the book would be very good. No, he did much more.

He knew from experience that heart disease is not lived alone, and he turned to his wife and caregiver for help. Then, from the caregiver's point of view, he spelled out all that it takes to live with the disease and how the caregiver is so intertwined in the recovery and the ongoing living process. In the sections from the caregiver, interspersed throughout the narrative, readers get advice as to what to expect and what they need to do. Recovering from and living on is a family affair, and Donna Selkow points this out in a friendly, caring, and understanding manner.

I found his approach to the subject to be extraordinary. Warren drew a metaphor using a three-legged stool to explain how cardiac care requires adherence to a complete program of diet, medications, and exercise. He convincingly makes the point that by not complying with all three legs of the stool, the foolhardy patient defeats the positive effects of the other two legs.

Warren has meticulously researched the book and provided attribution in the form of footnotes. He tells you where he got the information and carefully separates opinion and observation from fact. Not content with doing this, he persuaded many doctors and other professionals to "vet" the book to ensure it includes no misinformation. He sought out and received help from a prominent cardiac surgeon, four cardiologists, two pulmonary specialists, four primary care doctors, three internists, two physical therapists, a psychologist, a behavioral analyst, a neurologist, two college professors of cardiology, a nutritionist, a clinical pharmacist, several nurses from different specialties and lastly, from other patients. Few works receive such scrutiny. If it is in the book, it is right.

The broad range of subjects covers the entire life cycle of coronary artery disease from first diagnosis, open-heart surgery when required, recovery from surgery, living through and past the ordeal, coping with the deleterious side effects, and setting a long-term lifestyle. What is most significant is the attention given to living for the long haul. New technologies will evolve improved cardiac treatment but the basic issues of how a patient must live will remain constant and unchanging; that is what is so unusual about this work.

In addition, Warren addresses even broader areas of concern by covering how heart disease affects other chronic diseases, most notably diabetes, chronic obstructive pulmonary disease, and renal failure. Although those sections are short and concise, he paints a clear picture of what is different and similar when patients suffer from more than one chronic disease.

This book is different from any other book ever written for the following reasons: (1) it is written entirely from a patient's point of view, (2) it covers how to live with the disease for a whole lifetime and not just for the first year or two, and (3) it provides the added perspective of a full-time caregiver.

If you have coronary artery disease or congestive heart failure or if you are the caregiver for a patient, this is must reading for you.

Dr. Joseph Caplan, Director of Cardiology Medicine, Banner Boswell Hospital and Banner Del E. Webb Hospital, Arizona, and CEO of Cardiac Solutions, Peoria, Arizona.

ᗣᕯᕮ

Warning:

This book is extremely blunt. It deals with the subject in a manner that some might find shocking. If you are easily offended by tense situations presented in a no-holds-barred manner, then do not read this book.

If you are suffering from or caring for someone with cardiac disease, this book will explain the situation, as it really exists.

Some reviewers found some of the material "shocking." Some reviewers did not like the tone of some of the material.

As the author, I maintain if someone is offended or finds this shocking, I am hitting the mark. If something I wrote offends you, I would suggest you look into yourself and ask why.

There is no gratuitous sex or violence in this book. I tried, but I failed.

Dedication and Thanks

Every book has a dedication. Every author, especially a first-time author, has to thank everyone in the (as my mother would have said) whole "gd" family. I am not a first-time author. I coauthored a business textbook. In the dedication for that book, I thanked the world.

This book is different. It is not a textbook. I have only one person that is deserving of my dedication.

To my wife and coauthor, Donna. This is the one person who was and still is with me through thick and thin, good and bad.

It is appropriate for me to thank many people. They are all those who took the time, patience, and care to vet the work. I have listed them on a separate page. The simple fact is this: without their kindness, dedication and direction this work would not have been as complete and as accurate.

∾

Professional Vetters

This book has been reviewed for medical accuracy, vetted and approved (listed in no particular order of importance) by:

Joseph Caplan, MD, Cardiologist, Cardiac Solutions, Peoria, Arizona; Medical Director of Cardiology for Banner Boswell Hospital and Del Webb Hospital, Sun City, Arizona

Robert Deutsch, MD, Internal and Pulmonary Medicine, Director of Respiratory Care, Alameda Hospital, Alameda, California

Shannon Valenzuela, MD, Board Certified, Pulmonary Medicine, Peoria, Arizona

Edward Kowaleski, MD, Internal Medicine, Medical Director Banner Arizona Medical Center, Peoria, Arizona

Darry Johnson, MD, Board-certified neurologist with Banner Arizona Medical Clinic since 1996; Medical degree from University of Kansas 1991; Neurology Residency and Fellowship from University of Arizona completed 1996. Stroke director Banner Boswell and Banner Del E. Webb Hospitals

J. Nilas Young, MD, Professor and Chief, Cardiothoracic Surgery, UC Davis Medical Center, Davis, California

Stephen Raskin, MD, Clinical Professor of Medicine, University of California, San Francisco; Chief Cardiac Graphics, Alameda county Medical Center, Oakland, California; Director Alameda Lipid Clinic, Alameda, California

Dr. Michael Cofield, Clinical Health Psychologist, specializing in Cognitive Behavioral Therapy working with the elderly, Banner Boswell Hospital, Sun City, Arizona and Banner Del E. Webb, Sun City West, Arizona

Michele Ridings, RN, Cardiac Disease Counselor, Cardiac Solutions, Peoria, Arizona

Ellen Webb, RN, BSN, CNOR, Tucson, Arizona

Leanne Kedzie, RN, CLNC, Banner Boswell Hospital, Peoria, Arizona

Mark Bank, MS, Clinical Exercise Physiology, Indiana University and Certified Exercise Specialist, American College of Sports Medicine. Supervisor of Cardiac Rehabilitation at Banner Boswell Hospital, Peoria, Arizona, and Banner Del E. Webb Hospital, Sun City, Arizona.

Rhonda James, RN, Clinical Manager, Cardiac Solutions, Peoria, Arizona

Barbara Vermillion, RN, CNOR, Transplant Coordinator, University Medical Center, Tucson, Arizona

Denise Wells, EMT, Anti-coagulation specialist, Cardiac Solutions, Peoria, Arizona.

Thomas Gregory Quinn, MD, Cardiologist, Oakland, California

Mark Nelson, MD, Internal Medicine, Cardiologist, Board Certified in Cardiology and Internal Medicine, Masters of Public Health, Certified Health Coach and Presidential Director: Take Shape for Life, Teaching and empowering people to create health in their lives. Troy, N.Y.

Mary Ann Zimmerman, Therapist, MC, LPC, Managing Director, Ultra Learning Systems, LLC and the Mindability Group, Peoria, Arizona

Mark Moeller, M.D. Family Practice Physician, Sutter West Medical Group in Davis, CA. Co-founder of MedHealthSolutions, a web-based company offering health behavioral change solutions for disease prevention and health optimization.

The conclusions, ideas, recommendations, and opinions expressed in this book, if not expressly attributed and documented either by text or footnote, are those of the authors who are solely responsible for content. The Vetters attempted to ensure that no gross misstatements of medical fact were expressed at the time of their review. The Vetters further made a good faith effort to ensure that nothing was put forth that contradicts general principles of sound medical advice. However, all content ultimately contained herein is at the discretion of the authors and not the Vetters. Further, no Vetter can be held liable for any information printed in this book. Lastly, the Vetters reviews of this book do not imply either explicit or implicit agreement with the opinions expressed.

ᐤᑌ

Preface

When I first started to write this, I had no plans as to what the final use of this book would be. In fact, it wasn't even a book. It was, at best, a short monograph. In the initial version, I was just going to report, as factually as I could, what I wanted to know and was afraid to ask when I first got sick. I thought then it was not necessary to tell my story; besides, readers would not appreciate it. I am not a doctor of medicine. Why should anyone listen to me? As you read this, you will decide if what I say has any worth.

As it turns out, it is very necessary for me to tell my story, but not all at once. That is boring and is just one old sick guy blowing off hot air. Instead, I will relate my experiences and what I remember. Someday we can all get together and swap tales of daring do about our shared experiences. Not! I have talked with many surviving open-heart patients. What is more important is helping you prepare for, accept, and live with the disease. Put that way it kind of sounds like living next door to overly loud neighbors. Not pleasant, but tolerable.

I gave that initial paper to my cardiologist with only the hope that he would find it worthwhile and give it to his patients. Things didn't work out that way. He came back and told me this was really about living with almost all chronic diseases and he named the big four: coronary artery disease, diabetes, renal failure, and pulmonary disease. I don't know squat about the last three of those diseases. However, the doctors do and they say that the advice I give in this book works for all the diseases. Who am I to argue?

I have firsthand experience in living with coronary artery disease (CAD) and, fortunately, none of the others. What the cardiologist told me is that millions of people suffer from both diabetes and CAD. This work could and would lessen the deleterious effects of those twin killers and allow the sufferers to live not only more comfortable and easier lives but longer lives as well. Shucks, Skippy, could I actually help others? It now seems so.

The conversation with my cardiologist, Dr. Joseph Caplan, CEO of Cardiac Solutions in Peoria, Arizona, started me to think about not only the day-to-day disciplines of CAD but also what the patient goes through starting with being diagnosed and then all the catastrophic events that ensue. I use the term "catastrophic," although, if you are diagnosed early on in the life cycle of serious cardiac disease, the term "life changing" might be more appropriate.

Actually, the conversation was with Michele Ridings, a registered nurse at Cardiac Solutions, who educates and treats patients with congestive heart failure and Hyperlipidemia (high cholesterol). Mrs. Ridings specializes in education and follow-up regarding diet and the other necessary life adjustments attendant on living with chronic heart disease. I do not recall exactly what Michele said but something in that comment triggered all this work.

I divided this book into four primary sections. The first section deals with preparing for and surviving open-heart surgery and the aftermath, and getting through the first six weeks after the surgery.

The second section deals with living with chronic heart disease for the long term. If you have already had open-heart surgery, then you may skip this first part and go right to either the aftermath section or the section about living with cardiac disease for the long haul.

The third section tackles the exacerbating circumstances of not only having heart disease but also diabetes, chronic obstructive pulmonary disease, and lastly, renal failure in multiple combinations.

The last main section addresses the psychological side effects of depression, anxiety, and stress.

As it turns out, the book is organized in pretty much exactly the order in which a patient lives with the diseases. Those who read and vetted the book recommended that all sections be read regardless of where a heart patient might be. Even those sections on the other diseases are helpful because of the additional information presented and the impact of those diseases on heart disease.

In my case, the long haul, that first heart attack turned out to be a blessing in disguise. If not for that heart attack, my condition would have gone undiagnosed, and in a few months, my heart would have literally exploded. It is understandable that most people would wish to never have a heart attack. This might actually fall into the category of "Be careful of what you wish for." The following story illustrates that point:

A man was born with a golden screw in his belly button. All his life he obsessed about that screw and all his life he tried to have that screw removed, all to no avail. That is until he met the ascetic guru from Nepal. He told this wise man of his problem and the wise man promised his wish would be granted if he followed the "way."

The man with the golden screw promised to follow whatever way was necessary if it would get rid of the golden screw. (Oh, how often we make promises without understanding the circumstances.) The guru laid out the plan to the man with the screw and off he went to follow the "way." The man with the screw went to the mountains of Nepal where he entered a Buddhist seminary and began a life of quiet contemplation and meditation.

For two years, he exactly followed the way until the day the guru came to him and said, "You are now ready." The guru directed the man with golden screw in his belly button to a high mountain and a cave at the summit. It took two days to climb that mountain and get to the cave. Inside the cave was a chest. Inside the chest was a note that read, "Fast for two days and then look back inside this chest."

Having come this far, the man with the golden screw in his belly button spent the next two days fasting. After the two days, he opened the chest and found another note that read, "Now spend one more day wishing as hard as you can for the screw to be gone and then look back inside this chest." Well, in for a penny, in for a dollar, as the saying goes, so the man with the golden screw in his belly button spent the next twenty-four hours wishing, as hard as he could, for the screw to be gone.

After the twenty-four hours, he looked in the chest and inside he found an envelope that read, "The answer for your quest lies within." Inside the envelope was a little gold screwdriver. The head of the gold screwdriver perfectly fit the slot of the gold screw in his belly button. No other screwdriver ever perfectly fit the head of the gold screw in his belly button. With great happiness, he turned the screwdriver and finally, after all the years of obsessing over that gold screw, the screw backed right out. Then his ass fell off.

Be careful what you wish for.

Caregiver notes: From time to time, it will be necessary to give some helpful advice and guidance to those providing care to the cardiac patient. Those paragraphs will be printed in italics, just like this.

All the caregiver notes come from my wife, Donna.

The caregiver should read the whole book, if for no other reason than to better understand what the patient will be living through. My wife, Donna, assisted me in writing the sections on the caregiver. And who better? She was with me through both open-heart surgeries and, frankly, I would not be alive today if not for her.

You will also notice much of the book is written in first person plural, we, a strange twist given there was only one sick person. Without my wife there would be no first person, I. We had to get through the serious sick times together. My wife, my primary caregiver, was with me step by agonizing step. My wife understood the grave nature of my illness, better than I did. I was living in Egypt on De Nile. Sorry for the horrible pun. Denial is a common side dish accompanying the diagnosis of serious cardiac disease.

When we first learned the seriousness of the diagnosis, I said, "Can't be." We are sure that many others have the exact same response. We sincerely hope you find some comfort in this book from learning you (the both of you) are not alone and you can both persevere and move on.

One last thought: Knowledge provides power, assurance, and survival. We are nine years post-op for the first open-heart surgery and seven years post-op for the second. We are also in better physical shape now than we were as far back as five years before the first surgery. What we say in this book works for us and it will work for you. Honest.

Special Authors' notes: The entire first section, that dealing with open-heart surgery, can scare the living bejabbers out of you. We were encouraged to either make the surgery section Part II or tone down the language. We carefully listened to the advice, considered how the information would fall on people, and then decided: Nah! We are not authors of scary movies and books. We do want to inform and help prepare. If I (as the patient) had known exactly what to expect and when to expect it, the first surgery would not have been so traumatic or fear laden. The second surgery was not the least bit traumatic in terms of fear. It hurt like hell, nonetheless.

The reviewers and vetters of this book all made a point of mentioning the amount of time given to caregiver notes.[3] The word "caregiver" did not even come into common usage of the English language until the early 1980s. It is important to make a distinction between caregivers and care providers. I want to make that distinction this: caregivers do not get the recognition for their work that care providers do. More often, people think of care providers in terms of "paid professionals." Caregivers, on the other hand, usually render their services as an act of love. This is a big difference. This is not to say that paid professionals are doing their work only for the money. Any person categorized as a "care" individual, to my way of thinking, answers to a higher calling. It is hard to minister to those sick and afraid, regardless of the circumstances.

Having said this, "caregivers" end up working in a more stressful environment. The caregiver usually lives with the sick individual and the care is a never-ending cycle of cleaning up, cooking, ensuring medication is taken on schedule, and a infinite number of tasks. In many cases, this goes on for years and years. We could not find the statistics, however, Dr. Mark Moeller[4] told us "burnout and depression rates have been studied and are known to be quite high among caregivers. Part of chronic and severe disease management is to screen caregivers for this." Worse, caregivers are usually not appreciated during the toughest of times of administering care. It is the nature of the beast.

---

3   **–noun**
    1.   a person who cares for someone who is sick or disabled.
    Origin:
    1980–85; CARE + GIVER
    Dictionary.com Unabridged
    Based on the Random House Dictionary, © Random House, Inc. 2009.

4   Mark Moeller, M.D. Family Practice Physician specializing in health optimization and disease prevention at Sutter West Medical Group in Davis, CA Primary Care Doctor, Sacramento California.

And one last disclaimer: We are not "medical people." We are just two average people, who at the age of fifty-eight found our lives turned upside down and inside out. We have had professional medical people vet all medical information for accuracy. Everything else we lived through.

Caregiver notes: Few people realize what the caregiver must live through. It is a physical and emotional gut-wrenching experience to get a loved one through open-heart surgery and then help the person deal with the disease. The long-term caregiver has to learn to live with the patient's disease as well as the patient does. The price of freedom is vigilance; to stay well will require you to stay vigilant. In the main text of the book, some statistics address life expectancy after heart surgery. They are enlightening. More importantly, those statistics demonstrate your importance, as the caregiver, to the long-term welfare and continuing good health of your patient. Please take those statistics to your heart.

It takes a team effort to stay well with serious heart disease. The team consists of your patient (the object of all the attention), the cardiologist for the regular monitoring of the disease, the cardiologist's medical staff for the maintenance of the disease, your general care physician, and other assorted folks that will come through on a regular basis. As the caregiver, you are the captain of the team. It will fall to you to ensure the proper advice is given and understood, and the patient follows instructions.

෴

Prologue or
How Did I Get Here?

Chances are you are reading this because of either suffering a heart attack that landed you in the emergency room or, after what was supposed to be a routine examination by your primary care provider, you got sent to a cardiologist. In either event, you are now under the care of a cardiologist. In my case, it was the emergency room route.

We explained in the preface how we came to write this book. We also explained why we felt it necessary to write all that we did. We spent a fair amount of time doing research to make sure we included no misstatements of fact. What we hadn't considered was what questions you need to ask your cardiologist as you move forward after your first visit.

Ten important questions to ask your Doctor about heart failure:

1. What is the likely cause of my heart disease and is there an underlying illness we can treat?

2. What is the severity of my heart failure?

3. What treatment options are open to me?

4. Is there a cardiac rehabilitation program to strengthen my heart that is open to me?

5. What treatment options are open to me if my symptoms suddenly get worse?

6. What lifestyle changes must I make to feel better?

7. How will my disease effect and affect my daily activities, such as having sex, playing golf, or babysitting my grandkids?

8. What changes must I make to reduce stress, anxiety, and depression.

9. How do I explain my disease to my friends, family, and coworkers? And should I bother?

10. Are there any clinical trials that I am prospect for and would they be of benefit?

We don't answer most of these questions in the text of the book. Those questions are outside our purview and are not the medical issues we set out to address. We do take on questions numbers 4, 5, 6, and to some degree 8. Somewhere along the way, you will need the cardiologist to answer all the above questions. The sooner you have the first of the many heart-to-heart (no pun intended) talks, the better prepared you will be. Do not be afraid to ask and, even more importantly, do not be afraid to hold the cardiologist's feet to the fire to give you complete answers. It is in the cardiologist's job description to keep you informed. There is one other route to this book. You may now find yourself in a position to be a caregiver to one you love. You will have more questions than the patient. Count on it. We will address all of your concerns in this book.

Just to recap about how we got to this point, here are the major causes of coronary artery disease listed in no particular order of importance:

- ✔ Genetics
- ✔ High blood pressure
- ✔ High Low Density Lipids[5] "bad" cholesterol
- ✔ Low High Density Lipids "good" cholesterol
- ✔ Menopause
- ✔ Not getting enough physical activity or exercise
- ✔ Obesity
- ✔ Smoking
- ✔ Diabetes
- ✔ Stress

∽

---

5 **Definition:** A lipid is a fat-like molecule that does not have the ability to dissolve in water and includes molecules such as cholesterol and triglycerides.
Lipids are one of the major building blocks of animal cells. Many times, lipids will be referred to as a "fat".
Also Known As: Fat

SECTION ONE –
"I HEARD THE NEWS TODAY,
OH BOY"[6]

---

6   **"A Day in the Life"** is a song by the British rock band, The Beatles, written by John Lennon and Paul McCartney, based on an original idea by Lennon. It is the final track on the group's 1967 album *Sgt. Pepper's Lonely Hearts Club Band*

As Yogi Berra[7] would say, "Before I tell you something, I have to tell you something." It is this: If you are reading this, you have probably been diagnosed with CAD in some magnitude of seriousness (maybe even requiring surgery) or, as in my case, CHF (as we so benignly call it). Your life did not just suddenly come to an end. <u>It has changed.</u> These coronary diseases are incurable. However, if you follow a few simple rules, you will be able to live a long time and, more importantly, with an improved quality of life with fewer miserable symptoms. All right, so maybe the rules are simple but living with the rules is neither simple nor easy. Now that I have told you that, I can begin to tell (as Paul Harvey[8] would have said) the rest of the story.

More than twenty million Americans are walking around with CAD. Coronary disease accounts for about twenty percent of all deaths. That equates to a daily death rate of five hundred folks just like you and me. Twenty percent of adults over sixty have coronary disease. If these statistics (as reported in the *New York Times*) were war casualties, which were not this bad in any war America has ever been involved in including the Civil War, there would be an immediate change of administration.

Coronary heart disease has a host of symptoms, which indicate degrees of seriousness. A common diagnosis is for an irregular heartbeat, called arrhythmia. Many times, this particular symptom is congenital in nature; in other words, you were born with it. In and of itself it may not be terribly serious, as people have lived long lives with it. My mother lived to be ninety-five and had an arrhythmic heart her entire life. We will write more about this later.

About the worst news you can get after being examined by a cardiologist is: "You need open-heart surgery

---

7　Lawrence Peter **"Yogi" Berra** (born May 12, 1925) is a former Major League Baseball player and manager.

8　**Paul Harvey** Aurandt, September 4, 1918 – February 28, 2009, commentator on the ABC Radio Network.

and I am sending you to Dr. Heart Surgeon." You may wonder what the difference is between the cardiologist and the heart surgeon. The answer is simple: hands. The cardiologist's principal function is to properly diagnose your condition, stabilize that condition, and, where possible and practical, provide therapies that foster regression. That is the key statement—where possible and practical, foster regression.

In the end, it will fall to the cardiologist to give you the instructions and care to keep you alive. The cardiologist will advise you about how to protect yourself against the threat of ongoing coronary blockages. This includes being watchful for the continuing development of atherosclerosis (hardening of the arteries), which can lead to future stroke, amputation, kidney failure, and future heart attacks.

The surgeon is the master mechanic that can repair the damage. This team approach has made open-heart surgery downright routine with extraordinary survival rates. Approximately 1,250,000 Americans a year experience, firsthand, just how well this team approach works. That is the number of open-heart surgeries performed every year in just the United States. I have no idea how many are performed worldwide but my guess would be over 5,000,000.

The surgeon provides the skill required when a mechanical fix is required; this means drugs and all other forms of treatment are not enough. To say simply that the heart surgeon is a master mechanic gives short shrift to the work. The training is long and arduous. The work is precise, demanding, and time consuming. Heart surgery is not done on a production line, nor is it done based on some preconceived idea of how long any given surgery will take. Your life will literally be in the hands of the surgeon holding the knife.

The decision to send you to a heart surgeon is not taken lightly. The cardiologist will have probably explored every other option and decided on surgery as a last resort. After exploring all the noninvasive diagnostic procedures (CT scan,[9] EKG,[10] chest X-ray, stress test, echocardiogram) and not being satisfied with the results, or the results indicate further study is required, the cardiologist will perform an angiography. This procedure inserts a tube through the femoral artery and runs it up into your heart. A dye is injected and an image is televised to the cardiologist. The doctor can see exactly how your heart is operating and if there are any blockages.

The good news about this procedure is the relative lack of discomfort. A patient is only mildly sedated and a local anesthetic is applied to the point where the small puncture will be made to insert the tube. Back in the day, this required an overnight stay. Now, with the new technologies, it is an outpatient procedure. You may not need surgery, as all that is required is a stent,[11] a device that is inserted through your artery and will keep the artery open. Lucky you. The procedure is not onerous and you will be back on the street in no time at all. Escaping surgery does not mean you can go back to all of your bad old ways. It does mean that you do not have to read all that immediately follows about going through open-heart surgery. Maybe you should read it and use the information to keep you on the straight and narrow in terms of taking care of yourself so you don't end up needing that surgery. Your choice— your heart is not beating in my chest.

---

9   Computed tomography, commonly known as a CT scan, combines multiple X-ray images with the aid of a computer to produce cross-sectional views of the body. Cardiac CT is a heart-imaging test that uses CT technology with or without intravenous (IV) contrast (dye) to visualize the heart anatomy, coronary circulation, and great vessels (which includes the aorta, pulmonary veins, and arteries). WebMD

10 An electrocardiogram (EKG or ECG) is a test that checks for problems with the electrical activity of your heart. WebMD

11 A stent is a mesh cage device that fits into the blood vessel that feeds the heart. The stent's purpose is to expand that vessel for easy blood flow. A stent is used when blockage is not severe enough to warrant surgery.

Let us face the situation that you cannot get by with a simple stent. We will begin the discussion with this: Congratulations! You are cordially invited to join the largest, nonexclusive, no dues or application forms required, "Zipper Club." This club is truly democratic, as the members come from all socioeconomic strata and have only one thing in common: the zipper-like scar running from the top to the bottom of the sternum, hence the name of the club. The motto of the club is: "Once unzipped you can never go back."

Caregiver notes: Your life as a caregiver begins immediately upon diagnosis. This diagnosis will be as hard on you as it is on your patient. In some cases, it will be even harder on you. There are basics to be being a caregiver. I list them here in no order of importance:

1. *Stay optimistic*

2. *Get educated*

3. *Have patience with the patient*

4. *Keep everything extra clean*

5. *Make tender loving care your stock in trade*

6. *Get help*

7. *Change your life philosophies and expectations*

8. *Get prepared*

9. *Stay the course*

10. *Exercise appropriate discipline*

At some point in the book, all the above will be explained. Most importantly, you must listen very carefully to exactly what the doctors are saying. As we move forward I will be making specific points as to what you must listen for and what you must take to heart.

General Background

You, as a patient or caregiver, are entering a world filled with new terms. Worse, most of the new terms will be rushed upon you, leaving you with little time to acclimate. This is not a desirable condition or situation. To help prepare you for the challenges, you need to understand a few basics of the background you will find yourself living in. In the next section, we will start with a discussion about measurements.

Measurement, Standards, Statistics, and Medicine

Once you are diagnosed with CAD, measurements will govern your entire life. Most people take this with a "grain[12] of salt" and never question just what all those measurements

---

12   **–noun**
   5. The smallest unit of weight in most systems, originally determined by the weight of a plump grain of wheat. In the U.S. and British systems, as in avoirdupois, troy, and apothecaries' weight, the grain is identical. In an avoirdupois ounce there are 437.5 grains; in the troy and apothecaries' ounces there are 480 grains (one grain equals 0.0648 gram).
   Origin:
   1250–1300; ME *grain, grein* < OF *grain* < L *gränum* seed, grain
   Dictionary.com Unabridged (v 1.1)
   Based on the Random House Unabridged Dictionary, © Random House, Inc. 2006

mean. They take it for granted the folks in the know understand just what all those numbers mean. I know I did. Here is a non-inclusive list of those things that will now be under close scrutiny:

- Weight
- Blood Pressure
- Cholesterol
  - Total, HDL, and LDL
- Drug Dosages
  - Efficacy and Tolerance
- Calories
- Organ Function
- Etc.

After reviewing the material in this book many times, I had a rude awakening. Even though I thought I knew what some of the many terms meant, I realized I had no idea how blood pressure is measured or what that measurement really means. I knew the difference between high and low blood pressure. I knew the difference between good and bad blood pressure. I even knew why the differences are important. What I didn't understand is what the basis of measurement is. I had to find out.

This led to the conclusion that I did not understand measurement as it applies to medicine. I spent a lifetime in the business world and I understand measurement as it applies to the health of a business. I know what it means when a mechanic tells me that my car tires require thirty-four pounds of air pressure or my gas tank requires eighteen gallons to be full and the car will go twenty miles per gallon in the city.

Most of us understand how temperature is measured. It is part of the physical world we live in and is based on physics. Temperature can be measured on at least three scales,

Kelvin[13] (which is the only measurement system capable of measuring absolute zero), Celsius,[14] and Fahrenheit.[15] You will receive temperature information depending on the country you are in. In most of the world, temperature is reported as Celsius. Here in the States, it is reported as Fahrenheit. Depending on where you are, the unit of measure is different.

The inventor of the thermometer figured out that a unit of alcohol would rise up a glass tube based on the amount of heat the tube was subjected to. The tube could be graduated and numbered. In fact, any numbering system you wanted to use could be assigned to the graduations. All that is important is that the user of the numbering system knows what the displayed results mean.

Obviously, this would not work with blood pressure. It is necessary to have a standard unit of measure that means the same to everybody. In the case of blood pressure, the inventor of the blood pressure cuff, the sphygmomanometer,[16] arbitrarily assigned the unit of measure. The inventor figured

---

13 The **Kelvin** is a unit increment of temperature and is one of the seven SI base units. The **Kelvin scale** is a thermodynamic (absolute) temperature scale where absolute zero, the theoretical absence of all thermal energy, is zero (0 K). The Kelvin scale and the Kelvin are named after the British physicist and engineer William Thomson, 1st Baron Kelvin (1824–1907), who wrote of the need for an "absolute thermometric scale." *Symbol:* **K**

14 Also, **Centigrade *pertains*** to or notes a temperature scale **(Celsius scale)** in which 0° represents the ice point and 100° the steam point. *Symbol:* **C**

15 **Fahrenheit** refers to a temperature scale that registers the freezing point of water as 32°F and the boiling point as 212°F at one atmosphere of pressure. *Symbol:* **F**

16 The word comes from the Greek sphygmus (pulse) and manometer, an instrument used for measuring the pressure of liquids and gasses. The sphygmomanometer was invented by Samuel Siegfried Karl Ritter von Basch and first appeared in doctors' surgeries in the 1880s. In 1896, Italian pediatrician Scipione Riva-Rocci introduced an easy-to-use variation of the sphygmomanometer that consistently gave reliable results. Harvey Cushing, recognized in the medical profession as the greatest neurosurgeon of the twentieth century, found Riva-Rocci's sphygmomanometer on a visit to Pavia in 1901 and soon popularized it.

out that the amount of pressure required to move blood through the body could be measured by seeing how much mercury could be forced up a glass tube. The blood pressure cuff was born. The numbering system was arbitrary; however, once established and adopted, the meaning of the results was known to all.

Indeed, all units of measurement are arbitrary in nature. All that is important is for the users of the metrics to agree and understand what the numbers mean. The scientists and medical people who created them assigned the metrics we will be dealing with in this work. The folks that invented the technologies got to determine the metric systems. The inventors determined something had to be counted and the inventors got to say what was being counted and how it was to be counted.

Just counting does not determine quality. It takes statistics to determine quality. To determine quality of results the inventors of the technologies had to run tests on large populations to determine what were good results and bad results. This takes time and costs lots of money. As regards body temperature, for example, the inventor of the thermometer did not wake up and say a well person has a temperature of 98.6 degrees. Many, many people had to have their temperatures taken to arrive at that number.

Body temperature, although constant in its definition of wellness, can be and is measured in different scales in different parts of the world. So is weight. Body weight is measured in stones, pounds, ounces, and kilos; your measurements conform to the system in place where you are.

This would not work for dosages of drugs. Dosages must be precise. How do they know how much to prescribe? We all know the expression "enough to kill a horse." The implied meaning is that whatever is being used is a lot. "A lot" has to be contingent on something and in medical parlance, that something is usually body weight. Usually, the smaller the body, the smaller the required dose.

There is one other determining factor. That factor is resistance to the drug. Everyone has a different tolerance level to drugs. Your body is always trying to achieve some balance between what you take in and how it will be used. Your body will also adapt to the drug and take steps to mitigate its effect. The undesirable result, at least in the case of narcotics, is both dependency on the drug and the requirement for continually increasing dosages.

How much is enough? While a drug is in development, the inventors conduct Food and Drug Administration-approved tests. It is during these tests that the issues of how much per each unit of weight, tolerance, body adaptability, and observable side effects are recorded and measured. Oh, I forgot to mention the most important factor: does the drug work and deliver the desired benefits?

To ensure a true standard of dosage, the world has adopted the metric system of measurement. It is hard to believe, but even here in the good old US of A, the metric system is the standard. Fluids are measured in liters, solids in kilos and grams. Medicine, like commerce, is global.

The concepts of your body trying to adapt and balance, body-weight-dependent dosages, and tolerance and dependency will become ever more important as this book goes forward.

These examples are true for all medical metrics. It is important you understand this fact. It is important for three reasons: (1) your life is going to be managed by the medical metrics, (2) it helps to understand why the numbers become so important in your diagnosis and treatment, and (3) why everything costs so much.

Metrics are gathered by defining the answers to only three questions:

1. How much

2. How many

3. How long

Knowing the answers to these three questions over time forms the basis for comparison. It is in the act of comparison that conclusions may be drawn. The conclusions form the basis of all diagnosis, which we will discuss in the next section.

From time to time, it is both informative and necessary to ask the doctor what the numbers mean. What is being counted and why this count is so important to you, as a patient. As will be stated often in this book, you are responsible for yourself. Knowing what the numbers mean and how they affect you is in the same category as being an informed consumer.

Measurement Mandates

Mandate 1: The inventors of the tests determine the measurements.

Mandate 2: All units of measurement are arbitrarily assigned.

Mandate 3: Measurement meaning is based on population testing results.

Mandate 4: Results of the measurement metrics are indicators of the patient's state of health.

Mandate 5: Medical metrics are universally understood.

Mandate 6: No single measurement determines the state of the patient's health.

Mandate 7: The greater the number of tests to gather the measurements, the more certain is the accuracy of the diagnosis.

Mandate 8: The greater the number of measurements taken, the greater will be the costs to be borne by the health care system and the patient.

Mandate 9: Without measurement, there is no basis of comparison and therefore there is no management.

Mandate 10: You get what you pay for.

Testing, Testing, Testing

Why is testing so important? The preceding section dealt with the development of metrics and measurement. That section set the ground rules for how your life will be measured. A more important question is "Why will your life be measured?" The simple answer would be, "Because it is necessary." This is not a very good answer. I had to give some serious thought to this and, frankly, I had to apply a lifetime of experience in business to come to a better conclusion.

What became apparent was the way medicine is practiced (here is that word I hate to use when it comes to medicine). Medical care has a life cycle, a beginning, middle, and end. An "end state" in medical care does not mean death. It does mean some predetermined goal has been achieved and the patient is in a maintainable and desirable condition. The word "desirable" is used advisably. The desirable may not be a "good" condition but it is the best that can be either expected or hoped for. Medicine does not promise miracles, although sometimes miracles are delivered.

The medical life cycle has six major phases and each phase has six aspects of interest. You can think of the life cycle as a grid of thirty-six boxes. Each box requires answers and most of the answers will come from some form of testing to develop the measurement metrics.

This is what that matrix looks like:

	What	How	Where	Who	When	Why
Referral						
Examination						
Diagnosis						
Treatment						
Observable Results						
Prognosis						

Each major phase, as demonstrated by the grid above, asks a set of interrogatives, which are the aspects. Each interrogative must be answered. No one box is any more important than any other box. What is important is if, as a patient, something is not working out well for you, something has been missed. For instance, if you are being treated and the treatment is not delivering the desired observable results, you can bet your booty that something serious has been missed in either the examination or the diagnosis.

Referral – addresses the issue of why you went to the doctor in the first place.

Examination – addresses all the issues of what and how some conclusion is going to be reached regarding what specifically is wrong. It is during this phase that most of the testing will be conducted.

Diagnosis – the reason for the examination is to get to a diagnosis, which many times may be an educated guess.

Without an accurate diagnosis you are in deep mud, just like the carter but without a god to call on for help.

Treatment – addresses how you will be cared for and what steps you, as a patient, must take.

Observable Results – addresses the effect of the treatment and if the desired end state is being achieved.

Prognosis – addresses the issue of long-term outcome and sets forth the essential follow-up routine that will make up the bulk of your remaining and ongoing medical care—in the case of heart disease and the other chronic diseases we will address, this would be the rest of your life.

Each step and each interrogative may have a set of tests required to answer the question, as Bugs Bunny would ask, "Eh, what's up, Doc?"

There are two types of tests: invasive and noninvasive. Most of the tests are noninvasive and these tests are routine in nature and performed on a very frequent basis. However, many tests require some form of invasive procedure and mandate either an overnight or short trip to a formal medical center.

The most frequent tests are the "vital signs", namely temperature, blood pressure, and pulse measurement. It seems these three measurements are made almost every time you turn around. The tests are the first indicators for all patients that something may be amiss. A sudden acceleration or deceleration of pulse on a continuing basis is not a good sign especially for a heart patient. Worse is when blood pressure takes a sudden jump or severe drop.

Blood testing is a never-ending quest for truth, justice, and the American way. The purpose of all those blood tests: to answer the question, "How is your body responding to all those drugs you are taking?" All drugs are toxic in nature and all drugs can have serious side effects. Among other things, the blood tests ensure your body organs—most notably your liver and kidney functions—are not being impaired. The tests are also to confirm adequate amounts of the prescribed drugs are in your bloodstream.

So what?

You can find the truth of it all very close to home and probably right at hand. Look at any prescription label and you will see all the following questions answered:

- **What** – The name of the drug you are taking
- **How** – The specific directions for taking the drug. Not only are you directed to take, as an example, one tablet three times a day, but you are given other instructions like take with food.
- **Where** – Two or more where questions are answered and they include at a minimum the address of the pharmacy and your address, plus the phone number of the pharmacy.
- **Who** – Two who questions are answered, including the name of the patient and the name of the doctor.
- **When** – Usually specific directions as to what times of the day you are to take the medication. This may vary when the patient is left to his or her own devices to decide the time to take a drug.
- **Why** – That most important question is never answered on the prescription label. However, the information sheet that comes with the filled prescription will have a statement explaining why the drug is usually dispensed.

Taking drugs is part of the treatment phase.

Every prescription issued in the United States must have all of the above information listed on the label. It is a USDA and FDA requirement. It is a law. There is no circumventing this law. This law is necessary for the protection of the public. However, the law adds much cost to the dispensing of every prescription, not the least of which is that very large container for a few pills. The size of the drugs does not determine the size of the container; the size of the label does.

Your life is going to be about maintenance, follow-up, and testing. Now you know that the most important of the "interrogatives," the "why" for all the issues, is what we will be discussing in this handbook.

Testing Truths

Truth One: Testing is mandatory and may be neither overlooked nor not done.

Truth Two: Not performing tests can lead to misdiagnosis or death.

Truth Three: With no testing, there is no measurement.

Truth Four: With no measurement there is no comparison, and with no comparison there is no conclusion.

Truth Five: Testing delivers the baseline metrics that constitute the answers to the interrogatives.

Truth Six: You can't learn about what you do not test for.

Truth Seven: The most important test is probably the one that was overlooked.

Truth Eight: You get what you pay for.

After all the testing and measurement, and usually in the diagnosis stage, the doctor will give you the news in the following ways:

- You have x and this is what we are going to do about it (this is called the definitive diagnosis). This might include sending you to a specialist. This is an acceptable situation.
- The testing indicates you might have x but we (you will notice doctors never talk in the first person when they are unsure and always talk in the first person when they are sure) need to do more testing. This is called the undecided diagnosis. Or, as stated under Examination, the educated guess.
- The testing is absolutely inconclusive and we need to do more tests. What this means is your doc does not know exactly what tests to have run and will revert to the attitude that it is better to run too many tests than too few.
- All the testing is inconclusive and I am recommending you to Dr. Y, a specialist. What your doc has just said is really, "Beats the hell out of me so I am sending you to some specialist that will charge you a lot more money but, I will not be liable for medical malpractice." This is a very acceptable option.
- It is a very good idea to have a primary care doctor do the complete workup prior to visiting a specialist. Specialists do not look at the big picture for your care. Specialists can miss life-threatening conditions because they are just not looking for them if those conditions are beyond the scope of their specialty.

How I Got To Meet the Surgeon or a Short History of *Stupidity*

In the mid 1980s, I awoke one night sweating and dizzy. My heart was beating very fast and I was mildly nauseous. Being a man, I ignored this. By the middle of the next day, I was feeling terrible and my heart still seemed to be racing. I acquiesced to my wife and went to a same-day clinic. Within minutes of seeing the doctor, I was sent to the nearest emergency room. I was suffering from atrial fibrillation. I was given drugs and in a short time, my heart returned to its normal beat. I was directed to go back to my primary care provider. Did I follow those instructions? Noooo

Several months later, I went to Washington to attend a porate meeting and to make some sales calls. I also plan to give a presentation to a major corporate client the follo ing week so I stayed in Washington over the weekend anc did some sightseeing. On Sunday morning, my heart startec the fibrillation again. Did you ever turn up at a Washington hospital ER on a Sunday? I don't recommend it. The ER was so busy we had to go out to a suburban hospital.

This time, I had to be put to sleep and shocked to get the heartbeat back to normal. I was instructed to go home and see my doctor. Did I do this? Nooooooo. I stayed and gave the presentation. Even my boss was starting to question my sanity. I brushed it all off as not being serious. Besides, I had too much to do to take any time off.

Sometime in the late 1980s or early 1990s, I was diagnosed with hypertension (high blood pressure) and high cholesterol. I went through a treadmill stress test. I failed that test but did not know it. Almost immediately after the test, I went off on a business trip, literally that very day.

Two days later my doctor caught up with me by phone while I was in New York attending an important corporate meeting (when you work for IBM every corporate meeting is important). "Warren," he started, "you failed the stress test, and we have to do an angiogram. We have already scheduled the appointment for the day after tomorrow so get home, immediately, and take it easy. No stress!" This news did nothing to improve the mood of my boss, who had directed me to give a management presentation the next day. No stress here. The call also did nothing to mitigate a newly elevated level of anxiety.

I gave the presentation, as scheduled. I never was very good at following a doctor's directions. I went home and the next day, I showed up at the appointed time and place. The test showed I had a blocked artery and I was held over a day so the cardiologist could try to clear the block with a catheter. No such luck. There was no recommendation for more invasive surgery and I did not know enough to ask.

Back I went to my internist. He prescribed drugs to lower my blood pressure and reduce my cholesterol; off I went into the world to pursue whatever it was I was chasing, now wearing the armor of the drugs. What a jerk I was.

I was the typical Type A personality hell-bent on self-destruction. Here is a partial list of the things I did not do:

1. Get my stress levels under control. Hell, man, I was supposed to be under a lot of stress. It was listed right there in my job description under my management duties.

2. Dramatically change my eating habits. Why should I change my eating habits? I was taking an anti-cholesterol drug so why did I have to be concerned? Besides, I needed all that food to keep my engine in high gear.

3. Exercise. I had never really exercised before so why should I start now? I honestly believed running through airports carrying bags, a briefcase, and an early laptop computer qualified as exercise. All that baggage was certainly heavy enough.

In effect, I did nothing right. And I got by with it, cheating myself, for several years. Now I have a question. Does any of this sound like you?

Heart disease, unless it is congenital, does not just start one day. In my case I had years of warning, all entirely unheeded.

The Surgeon

Your time with the surgeon is short, limited to an initial visit for what is best described as the "feel good" session. During this visit, the surgeon will explain what he or she will do and what your chances of survival are. These are necessary steps. You are going to be scared out of your wits, as you should be. The fear is rational and justified. There is much you do not know, and you are afraid of "the unknown." By the time you finish reading this first section, you will know the unknown. The only thing left is the hardest part, experience.

When you get to see the surgeon depends on three factors:

1. How your disease is discovered

2. How severe your disease is

3. How much time you have to be saved

Many patients find out how sick they are when the cardiologist does the angiography. The disease is already so far progressed the patient really cannot afford to leave the hospital. This is an emergency situation. And speaking in terms of an emergency, there is always the possibility of a heart attack where the patient winds up in the emergency room holding on to dear life by a thin thread. There is generally not much time for careful consideration of the options. You may not even get to have any conversation with the surgeon. You wake up when it is all over.

In many cases, if not most, the surgery, although absolutely necessary, is not an emergency. Some time may elapse for the patient to prepare for the surgery. In the non-emergency but necessary example, your next visit with the surgeon is likely to be the morning of the surgery while you are in the "prep room." The surgeon will reassure you that all is well and you will next visit after the surgery. The surgeon rarely keeps this promise, but that is all right. After surgery, when you wake up, you will be in the hands of a group of professionals who really know their stuff. Rest assured, you will be in good hands. Your last visit with the surgeon will be one last follow-up to ensure all the "i's" are dotted and all the "t's" are crossed, etc. Then you will return to the care of your cardiologist, and not a minute too soon.

Depending on the circumstances of your condition, several other steps would be appropriate:

- A trip to the hospital where the surgery will be preformed is a smart thing to do.
- A blood clotting test to determine the speed with which your blood clots.
- A meeting with your primary care nurse who will be waiting for you when you open your eyes.
- A tour or orientation of the cardiac intensive care unit (CICU).
- A booklet, written for morons, not intelligent people like you, describing what to expect. In retrospect, the booklet was downright misleading.

Having been through this more than once, one other very important step is suggested: get your teeth cleaned and any cavities filled before the surgery. There is a direct bloodline from your heart to your teeth. Having your teeth cleaned and repaired prior to the surgery eliminates one potential for unwanted infections. And don't forget to take the antibiotic prior to the dental work. Dentists will make room for you in their schedules when you explain you are going to have open-heart surgery and need to see them immediately. (Since writing this a change has occurred. Doctors may no longer prescribe antibiotics for all patients with valve disease. If your cardiologist or doctor recommends antibiotics, take them.[17])

Get a haircut. You are not going to feel like getting a haircut for six or seven weeks so get one before the surgery. You'll thank me later for this.

Here is the very best advice we can give you for after your diagnosis: go with the flow. You will have two options. One, you can do nothing and die. Two, you can accept what is about to happen and let it just occur at its own pace. If you are not going to make a concerted effort to change your nasty ways and take it all with the degree of seriousness the illness demands then, by all means, select option one.

Caregiver notes: One of the main problems with this process is the rapidity of the events. You get little or no time for careful consideration of the options. No time is available when the situation is an emergency. The medical profession can take no time to consider if the surgery will be worthwhile. The patient and the patient's family have no time to discuss what change will have to be made. Nope, there is the mad dash to get the person into the operating theater and crack open that chest.

---

17   Dr. Mark Nelson, Cardiologist and Dr. Mark Moeller, Family Practice, Davis, California

One of the more deleterious effects of this process is the introduction of a high degree of fear into all concerned. They really lay on the fear, as if just the weight of the bad news is not enough. My guess as to the reason for the great fear burdening is to communicate the seriousness of the problem.

From my perspective as a wife and caregiver, it would have been very helpful to go through a couple of other steps. These are some things that would have made life a lot easier:

- Education detailing dietary changes
- Education about the drugs to be administered
- Education about the lifestyle changes
- Education about the exercise requirements
- Education about what will be expected of the caregiver
- Education about what the responsibilities of the patient will be

Another thing you will quickly notice as a caregiver is a complete change of attitude on the part of your patient. Fear will cause many personality changes, none of them for the good. The changes are almost immediate upon diagnosis. You will also notice some changes in yourself. Here are the warning signs:

- Shortness of patience
- Irritability at almost everything
- Guilt (all of which is a waste of time)
- Defensiveness
- Nastiness
- Depression

The doctors will spend some time on certain areas, given the seriousness of the situation and how fast the surgeons want to move. But mostly, the surgeons just want to move fast. Maybe they have a late tee time. Sorry, unfair shot. The cardiologists will spend some time explaining the nature of the emergency, the nature of the heart disease, and why they have to hurry the hell up. My patient had a completely shot aortic valve, a seriously malfunctioning mitral valve, four completely blocked lines, and an aneurism on the aorta the size of a golf ball. He had a greatly enlarged heart. We did not rush into surgery. We delayed two weeks. Think about your situation before you sign any consent forms.

After careful consideration, I have decided to broach this subject here instead of later on. It deals with alcohol use. I am not passing any judgment here. Many people use alcohol on a regular basis. Both the cardiologist and the heart surgeon must know this and it will probably be left to you to clue them in. Heavier users will have serious problems during recovery and the medical staff absolutely must know. To be blunt, if the patient is an alcoholic there is a good chance during recovery of hallucinations, incoherence, and even death if the physicians caring for the patient do not know to give the appropriate medications to prevent a withdrawal. An informative word could save a life.

Before going any further, it is necessary to give you some bad news/good news. We like to get the bad news out of the way first. The bad news:

- Open-heart surgery hurts like hell. Your sternum has been sawed in half and until that bone knits about five to six weeks after surgery, every breath you take can be agony.
- You will be afraid. This may sound silly, but do not be afraid of being afraid.

- Open-heart is massively invasive and your body does not like that, so you will suffer a number of other complications, not the least of which is depression. You will also be Stressed with a capital S. We will deal with both of those subjects in detail later.
- The wounds left immediately after the surgery are both ugly and frightening. Veins harvested from legs and arms for grafts for bypasses leave ugly wounds that require lots of stitches. As the saying goes, "That's going to scar."
- Some will tell you the doctors technically kill you to do open-heart. With friends like this, you need no enemies. This is not so. You may be placed on a heart-lung machine. This machine will keep you alive quite nicely, thank you, while the surgeons are doing their magic.[18]

One more thing before we move on. Nothing is going to happen until the medical system knows how you are going to pay for all that is about to happen. Open-heart surgery is very expensive. Oops, sorry, we weren't supposed

---

18 **Cardiopulmonary bypass (CPB)** is a technique that temporarily takes over the function of the heart and lungs during surgery, maintaining the circulation of blood and the oxygen content of the body. The CPB pump itself is often referred to as a *heart-lung machine* or *the pump*. Cardiopulmonary bypass pumps are operated by allied health professionals known as perfusionists in association with surgeons who connect the pump to the patient's body. CPB is a form of extracorporeal circulation.
Dr. Clarence Dennis led the team that conducted the first known operation involving open cardiotomy with temporary mechanical takeover of both heart and lung functions on April 5, 1951, at the University of Minnesota Hospital. The first successful open heart procedure on a human utilizing the heart lung machine was performed by John Gibbon on May 6, 1953, in Philadelphia. He repaired an atrial septal defect in an eighteen-year-old woman.

to mention that part. Well, the cat is now out of the bag. Deal with it.

Caregiver notes: This might sound cold and uncaring, but not everyone that needs open-heart surgery should have it. If the patient is not willing to make the changes that will be required, why go through the pain and aggravation and why put the family through the grief and expense? It only prolongs the time until death, not the eventuality of death; it's only a matter of how long and how much suffering is going to go on until death occurs.

From firsthand experience, I have seen many people who should not have gone through the agony of the surgery. In no less than ten cases, and probably more, the people survived the surgery only to die within the next year. Worse, from my perspective, their quality of life had deteriorated so much that they spent that year in deep depression and constant pain.

In one very hard-to-watch scenario, the husband had open-heart surgery. He had spent his whole life depending on his wife for virtually everything. She stepped up to the bar and took on the duties of caregiver. A year or so later, she needed open-heart surgery. She had no one to be her caregiver so she had to be the caregiver for both of them. She died within three months of her surgery. He died three weeks later.

Senior citizens advancing in age, should not, in my opinion go through the hell of the experience. If the support network is not really in place and if the patient is very set in his or her ways and cannot or will not make all the changes required, then don't do it. This is just my opinion.

This subject of finances is so important to the care and well-being of the patient and the caregiver that we will address it right now. We will address finances again but some comments are in order right now. Once the ball gets rolling on the medical issues, attention can move off the financial issues.

Somebody is going to have to ensure all the money concerns are addressed and there is always the chance the patient will not be able to be responsible. It is imperative that proper controls and help are in place before the surgery, if possible. Not only is this important for a spouse but children may be called on to help. As we age, our children are going to be expected and called upon to step in and look after the estate. This is a big responsibility and duty.

There are a few guidelines:

- The trustee must be someone that can be trusted with money.
- The trustee must understand the wishes of the patient and the family.
- The trustee must be responsible.
- If a family member does not fulfill the above three items, get a professional to help.

Few things in the world can tear asunder a family faster than the requirement for a sick parent's care and the care and control of the finances. This is sad, but it is true.

This next part is very hard. The survival rate for open-heart surgery is ninety-six percent. Only four percent of all those that undergo this surgery do not survive. There are many reasons for not surviving. Here is a list of some of those reasons:

- The patient is severely de-conditioned (too obese, too out of shape, no physical reserves due to other illness, longtime smoker, excessive drug or alcohol use, etc.)
- The surgery is too great a shock to the system.

- *The patient was not really a candidate for the surgery but decided to go through with it anyway (remember surgeons are compensated for doing the surgery, as is the hospital, and not for the long-term outcome and welfare of the patient).*
- *The patient did not want to have the surgery but did it to satisfy family demands.*
- *Very, very rarely, the surgeon blunders or some other unfortunate event occurs in the operating room. This is generally the last cause of death and the least significant.*
- *The patient did not seek care soon enough and the cardiac disease is in a very advanced state.*
- *The patient ignored all the warning signs and has had a catastrophic heart attack.*
- *The patient just does not want to survive.*

If you find yourself wondering if the surgery is worth the pain, aggravation, and grief, then some would conclude not to bother. Death is bad enough without prolonged suffering. Prolonged suffering and torture are the same thing.

The death of a loved one is a hard thing to face and accept. Accepting the reality is made even harder when, as caregiver, you must take care of the patient every day and watch the suffering. It is very difficult to be upbeat for the patient while you are crying inside. Yet this is exactly what you must do. In my life, I have had to care for several terminally ill family members. I do not have all the answers nor can I give the very best advice. No one knows what the very best advice really is. Every situation is different.

There are two things you can do if you know there are long odds against survival. The first thing you can do is to tell your loved one you love him or her. This is very important for both you and the sick person. Telling of your love provides affirmation for the patient. In our lives it is very important to love and be loved. Hearing the words "I love you" provides reassurance. In your whole life were those words ever inappropriate or unwelcome when said to you? In your whole life when you said those words to the person you love, were they ever rejected?

The second thing you can do is say, "Good-bye." This simple word will help provide closure. When my loved ones were in their final days I always made it a point of saying, "I love you," and, upon parting, "Good-bye."

And now the good news:

- You are going to live and you are going to feel a whole lot better after the surgery. This is so important, it bears repeating: YOU ARE GOING TO LIVE AND YOU ARE GOING TO FEEL A WHOLE LOT BETTER AFTER THE SURGERY! Did you get that? No? OK: YOU ARE GOING TO LIVE AND YOU ARE GOING TO FEEL A WHOLE LOT BETTER!!
- You will receive drugs that will mitigate the pain. The drugs will keep you in a dream state for several days, which you will welcome, believe me on this.
- You won't remember much about the total experience. This is the result of one particular drug—a hypnotic that blocks out all the bad stuff going on around you. No memory, no pain. Wonderful. The effect of the drug will extend from before the surgery until well after

it. In my case, I remember that it all hurt, but I don't remember why. There is comfort in this. The most disconcerting effect in my case was that it clobbered my short-term memory. It took some time before I regained full use of my vocabulary.

Now for some even better news:

- Your cardiologist is going to help you get back on your feet faster than you have any right to expect.
- There is a large support network, not the least of which is the "visiting nurse" system. This is good news.
- The only caveat to this is you must be willing to cooperate and follow instructions.
- Believe it or not, the open-heart surgery event is going to be the easiest part of the whole experience of living with chronic heart disease. For the surgery, you need only be passive. That will all change.
- The patient is part of a "team." By being the most active participant of the team, you—the patient—will heal not only faster, but also better. One of the more important aspects of the post-op treatment is the spirometry treatment. The spirometer is a device that measures your lung output. It is a painful exercise, in the beginning, but it is an important measurement of your continuing improvement. The nurses will need you to try hard and get off your ass, even with the pain.

Caregiver notes: As the in-home caregiver, you will be in charge of ensuring compliance with all the rules. It will not be easy. Some of those rules take effect immediately following diagnosis.

Your patient can become rather hard to deal with. Your patient is going to have to give up control of everything and is likely to resent it, especially if your patient is a Type A personality like my patient. And if your patient ever had a tendency to be disgruntled and nasty, this event will bring it all out.

The Big Day Arrives

Depending upon the severity of the disease, the amount of time you have, the hospital, and the time of day surgery is scheduled for, the following instructions will probably be issued to you:

- The night before the surgery, you will probably be asked to shave your chest from neckline to waist. The incision will be from slightly above the sternum to well below it. You may also need to shave your legs from groin to ankle. This is the first candidate location for vein harvesting. The number of bypasses required will determine the number of different locations the veins will be harvested from.
- You will be given a strong antibacterial soap to wash with. Scrub well.
- You may have nothing to eat or drink for at least twelve hours prior to checking into the hospital for surgery. Obey this instruction. The last thing you want is to be vomiting as soon as you wake up.

- Take no jewelry, watches, rings, necklaces, or any other adornment to the hospital. The hospital will not want to be responsible for those items.
- Wear as few clothes as possible and only those things that you will want to wear home after the event.
- If you wear removable bridgework or false teeth, leave them home. Your spouse can bring them to you when you are able to eat. You will not be able to eat for at least two days after the surgery. You will not feel like it.
- If you require a hearing aid, take it with you; the same for spectacles. You will want them when the time is appropriate.
- The hospital will probably want you there at least one to two hours before surgery. You will be checked in and the billing will begin.
- In the surgical check-in area, someone will take you to a preparation area, give you a gown, and tell you to strip and don the gown. A nurse will take your things and put them in a bag that will follow you through the process.
- Take no valuables of any kind.
- The prep nurse will take your vitals. Your vitals are going to be taken hundreds of times in the next few days.
- The prep nurse will run the first of the many lines you will be receiving in the next few hours.
- You will take a tranquilizer to start the sedation process. You will meet the doctor who will be charged with keeping you asleep during the procedure. The doctor will explain what drugs you will be receiving to keep you asleep.
- All the medicines enter your system through the intravenous lines.

- At the appropriate time, you will say good-bye to whomever brought you to the hospital and someone will wheel you to the cardiac operating theater.
- You will move from your gurney to the operating table.
- You will not experience any sense of panic and you will be amazed at how calm you are.

Your gown will be removed and you will be covered to keep you warm. There will be many people in that operating room. They might tell you what their jobs are. It will make no difference to you. In a few minutes, you will be asleep. You will be told to start to count down from one hundred. You will not make ninety and even if you do, you will not remember it.

Contrary to your belief, the cardiac surgeons are not the most important people in the room. It is the anesthesiologist. That doctor is the one keeping you alive and unconscious. Once you are asleep, it makes no difference to you what is happening. You need only believe you will be waking up after it is all over and you are going to be better for the rest of your life.

The health care system has made a huge investment in education for the professional staff attending you, equipment, and supplies to ensure the best chances for your recovery and survival. We wondered just what the typical investment might be for a "simple" bypass procedure. I asked Dr. J. Nilas Young[19] for a list of what is on hand for such a "typical" operation.

This is what he had to say: **"There are approximately nine people involved in the surgery—an anesthesiologist, an assistant, three surgeons (one may be a physician assistant or resident), three nurses, and one perfusionist**

---

19   J. Nilas Young, MD, Professor and Chief, Cardiothoracic Surgery, UC Davis Medical Center, California

(heart-lung machine technician). The equipment in the OR is vast and I really shouldn't task someone with listing it. It involves approximately one heart-lung machine, one anesthesia machine (with ventilator), an echo machine, probably at least three EKG/blood pressure monitors, over one hundred surgical instruments, and, of course, a small room next to the OR with a million bucks worth of valves, sutures, and various other disposable/one-use instruments."

What is not on this list is what you cannot see. Behind this "front line," so to speak, is a literal army of professionals whose sole purpose is to get you through this experience and on your feet to lead the rest of your life—not to mention the huge investment in equipment that is also essential to your care and recovery. Nobody that cares for you will have had less than two years of formal education, and most will have had at least four years of education and training. They will all be either board certified or state certified in their fields of care. There is no on-the-job training for these professionals.

If you were wondering why open-heart procedures are so expensive, now you know.

New technologies are at work in how the operation is performed. It is now not always necessary to stop the heart and use the perfusion technology. New advances have figured out how to stabilize that section of the heart to be worked on. The heart is never stopped. How the surgery is performed is contingent on the severity of the disease.

Remember, the less the surgeon has to do, the less severe the shock to the system, the shorter the hospital stay, and the shorter the recovery time.

Caregiver notes: Stay with your patient until the last minute. Learn what is going to be happening. This will be comforting to you. Knowledge is both power and reassurance.

Getting Your Eyes to Work

Waking up after the surgery is a shock to the system all its own. When you wake up, all the following will be true:

- Happy April Fools' Day. You are alive and awake. Or awake and alive, take your pick. And it hurts. I start this list with this comment because I have learned that some who opt for this surgery really do not wish to get through it. Strange, huh? Not really. Some people live their lives as if there is no tomorrow so when they have the big heart attack it is just the price to be paid for the excess. Well, tough luck for you, then, Bunky. Thanks to good technology, good doctors, and just plain dumb bad luck, you are still here. Now you will get to learn the price to be paid for your stupidity, just like I did. Ha, ha, ha, ha.
- There will be a tube in your mouth. This is a respirator tube that will assist you in breathing. This is very necessary, even if it is frightening. The professionals will get this tube out of your mouth as soon as they are satisfied your lungs work on their own.
  - They will ask you to cough as soon as the tube is pulled. This is to expel any sputum in your breathing passage. This hurts. Hold onto and grasp a pillow tightly to your chest before coughing. This helps. You are going

to need the pillow a lot so keep it handy. Should I mention laughing also hurts?

- Your hands are going to be restrained. When you wake up you will be confused and your first inclination will be to pull the lines that are sticking into more places than you want to count. The restrained hands prevent this.
- You may experience some degree of panic and strain against the restraints. Don't bother. Stronger people than you have tried to no avail.
- Waking up in this alien world will make you fearful. If you are afraid, you are having the right reaction.
- You will probably immediately notice the beep, beep, beep of all the monitors attached to you. You are in good shape as long as those monitors keep a regular beeping sound.
- There will be a full-time dedicated cardiac nurse right outside your door, twenty-four hours a day for the first several days. That nurse is monitoring everything that is happening to you, and has no responsibilities other than your immediate welfare and care.
- You will have to be pulled up in your bed on a regular basis. Although this can be painful, it is necessary, so go with the flow.
- You will be thirsty when you get the tube out. You will not be given anything to drink. You will be given ice chips to suck. The nurse will tell you when you can have more. Suffer it and go with the flow.
  - So what happens if you do drink something? You will throw it up, almost as fast as you drank it. Throwing up hurts.

- You will have drain tubes coming out of your chest and these tubes will be pulled. This hurts and feels like you are being pulled over a washboard. But it is fast and quickly over with.
- You will have a urinary catheter so don't worry about getting out of bed to use the toilet.
- You will be wired to a pacemaker that ensures a steady heartbeat. These wires will also be pulled out. I don't remember this hurting.
- Every morning at 3:00 a.m. X-ray techs will awaken you when they come to take a new chest X-ray. This is particularly exasperating. The last place you can really get any sleep is in a cardiac intensive care unit, or CICU. It is very noisy. So just when you can get to sleep, these folks come in and tell you to roll over so they can put the film under your back. It is very hard to get back to sleep. The techs take the X-rays when they have the most time available to take the pictures; the docs need them for their 8:00 a.m. rounds.
- About the issue of noise—it is very noisy on the CICU. Some hospitals call this a surgical intensive care unit. There are lots of machines and lots of people scurrying to and fro. Strongly request ears plugs. Do not accept the "We do not have them" answer. You may have to insist and you should do just that. Bitch, bitch, bitch—sometimes it is the only way. Realistically though, you may have to take your own or have someone go buy them for you. This is very important. Sleep in the immediate time following the surgery is very essential. Take it from this trooper the CICU is noisy, it can't be helped.

- A vast army of residents and interns will visit you, all checking your vitals and all standing around talking about you in the third person. I asked if they had forgotten I was in the room. All I received for that query was a blank look.
- You will probably be wearing a pair of elastic stockings. The stockings help cope with the edema that usually occurs in the legs and ankles. You will be wearing these stockings for many weeks after the surgery.
- The food you eat will taste like boiled card-board. You will be put on a no-sodium, no fat, no-taste, no-caffeine, and no-texture diet. This will make you wish you were dead. You will lose real weight, and you won't even have to try hard. Some patients gain weight but it is water weight and you will soon be given a diuretic to get it off. Your appetite will be depressed for months, especially once your caregivers tighten the reins on your eating habits. I sure hope you like warm gelatin dessert. I ate a lot of graham crackers. I now hate graham crackers.
- It is of paramount importance that you choke down as much of the food as you can. Nutrition is important to the rapidity of your healing.
- What you eat, thanks to the pain relievers, will make you constipated.
- Start to demand stool softeners and drink as many fluids as you possibly can. You are going to have to move your bowels before you get to the next phase of care and without those stool softeners, it will be very painful and diffi-cult. Your inability to move your bowels will also generate a tremendous headache, which will be treated with more pain relievers.

- Make damn sure your cardiologist is prescribing all this stuff for you. If you want to get ahead of the curve on this, use this total list as a prompt and guide. Have the cardiologist sign off on the list.
- Forewarned is prepared. If I had my way, which I don't, I would make this list mandatory for every cardiac patient. Mental preparation is just as important as physical preparation.
- You are going to be an unreasonable jerk with your loved ones. You will deserve it if they never speak to you again as long as you live after you get out of the hospital. The first thing you are going to have to do is apologize to everyone for being such a schmuck.

Caregiver notes: Prior to the surgery, your loved one will need tons of emotional support. The soon-to-be surgerian or surgeree (words we have just now made up) will be frightened. The fear can come from two areas: (1) the fear of death; and (2) the fear of what will happen to you, the remaining spouse or other close loved one, if the surgery fails and death ensues. To prevent this fear from becoming all consuming, there are some things you can do:

- *Help ensure all the affairs are in order. (We had to do this the first time around. This included making a will, setting up a trust to avoid probate, and signing a medical power of attorney and a financial power of attorney [two different documents and both necessary].) The benefit of this step delivers some peace of mind. Also, once it is done, it is done.*
  - *The medical power of attorney, also called an advanced directive, is very important.*

The patient might reach a state when making a rational, sound decision is not possible. After the second open-heart surgery the docs suggested a pacemaker to ensure a steady heartbeat. My patient said no to this idea; he would rather stick with the wonderful drugs. Exercising the advanced directive, I overrode this wrong-headed decision and a pacemaker was implanted that very day. What he did not understand at that time was his suffering from sleep deprivation. What made this apparent was his response to the question, "Where are you?" He said to the doctor, "I am in Boston to see the Kennedys." I stepped right in and ordered the pacer.

- *Give constant reassurance the patient is going to be all right.*
- *Give constant reassurance that you are going to be there.*
- *Give constant reassurance the patient has good, competent doctors who will provide quality care.*
- *Give constant reassurance that if the worst happens, you and the family will be all right.*
- *Accompany the patient to all the preoperative tests and visits.*
- *Actively question the doctors as to the facts, and make sure the patient hears you are taking an active role in the recovery.*
- *Begin the required regimes and start to exercise the discipline that will be necessary for the patient's recovery.*
- *Be proactive in the patient's education.*
- *Forget about the laying on of guilt with recriminations. The last thing a patient wants to hear is somebody saying to him or her, "I told you so."*

- *Never, for one moment, exhibit any fear to the patient. This is extraordinarily difficult but extraordinarily important. You may break down and cry two to three weeks after the surgery, when the patient has turned into a first-class pain in the ass.*
- *Remember this above all else—recovery begins immediately with diagnosis.*
- *Since recovery begins with diagnosis, get your patient on the appropriate diet. If nothing else, have your patient start eating at least five fresh fruits and vegetables a day.*
- *Take a good multivitamin. You want to have as many reserves as possible in your body. Oh, and have the patient take one too.*

Immediately after the surgery, your role as caregiver is going to drastically change. And you will have to face another set of serious challenges. Your first challenge has to do what to do with yourself during the surgery. I don't advise hanging around the waiting room. The surgery can take anywhere from six to twelve hours, and in extreme cases, even longer. The first open-heart took thirteen hours, but the patient was a really sick puppy. My son and I went home until someone called and said my husband was in the CICU and awake.

This is what you can expect when you show up at the CICU:

- *Put on a brave face. You are going to walk into a room filled with beeping machines, your loved one will be tied down, and there will be a tube stuffed down the throat. It will look uncomfortable and it is.*

- *You may be afraid. You are entering a surreal alien world. You must act like the experience is completely normal and everyday.*
- *Start by saying, "Welcome back. See, I told you (this is the only time the expression 'I told you so' is permissible) everything would be all right. The doctor says you did just fine and everything is proceeding on schedule." I cannot stress too strongly the need for this reassurance.*
- *Spend as much time as you can in the room. In the CICU there is a certain degree of laxity as to visiting hours. Family support is important to recovery. Don't worry if the patient is cognizant of your comings and goings. The patient is not going to remember much of the first few days after surgery. Bless those drugs.*
- *After three days, if all is going well, your patient will be moved into the cardiac care unit. This is a good sign. Of course, the patient won't see the nurses as much but then the patient doesn't need to.*
- *In five or six days, your patient is going home.*
- *For the first few days after surgery, it is not unusual for your patient to be nasty as hell. Your patient may be verbally abusive to you but very nice to the professional staff. This is unreasonable and hard to take. However, this is not your fault and you may not and cannot take ownership of the situation. What is at work here is a "reverse effect." Your patient is lashing out at the situation and not you. Here are the causes for this strange turn of events:*
  - *Drugs.*
  - *Your patient may have a self-image of being your "knight in shining armor" and*

> *the serious surgery is tarnishing the self-image.*
>
> · *Up until right now, your patient has been in total control and now has no control of anything. Remember the nurses are making the patient do things they do not want to do, like get on their feet and walk.*
>
> · *Pain and discomfort can cause the nicest person to turn into a monster.*
>
> · *Your patient might really be a nasty jerk and you just never noticed it before.*
>
> • *Your patient is not in control of his or her behavior right now and the answers are inappropriate.*
>
> • *You should seriously consider putting your patient in a short-term care facility until the old attitude comes around. You may not do anything that will put your own health in jeopardy. It makes no sense for your patient to live by killing you.*
>
> • *Your patient may also be sullen or withdrawn and treat you with silence.*
>
> • *When your patient gets sassy and demonstrates an attempt at being funny, rest assured healing is taking place.*

Out of the CICU and into the CCU

About three days after surgery, you will probably be well enough to be moved from the cardiac intensive care unit and into the cardiac care unit (CCU). This is a big step down in care. You will miss all those people running around. You will also have a roommate. Tough. You will want to share experiences. Don't. Your roommate probably will care as much about what you have just come through as you will really care about what your roommate has come through.

What this really boils down to is bragging rights as to who was sicker. You will have many people you can bore with your tales of terror and horror, but this roommate is not one of them. Besides, you are never going to see this person again. In short order you will believe your roommate is a complete dumb cluck. What do you think family is for? They are the ones you can bore the daylights out of. Family is obliged to nod and say, "Poor baby."

Life in the CCU is more normal, if life in a hospital can ever be described as normal. The meals will come on the same ugly trays with the same boiled cardboard. The routine will be very different. For one thing, not so many machines. Most of the machines will be at the nurses' station and you will be wired up for transmission. The nurses on this ward are not as sympathetic as the CICU folks. They have seen lots of sickies, many a lot sicker than you.

You are going to be told in no uncertain terms to get your butt out of bed and to join the brigade of "bare butt marchers." There is no fighting it. You are going to have to get immediately mobile. Face up to it, grab your IV pole, cover your bare butt as best you can, and get walking around the halls of the unit. Think of it as a waltz. Push the pole, take two steps. Push the pole, take two steps. All together now: push, step, step, push, step, step, push, step, step. You got it. Now you're doing the Cardiac Rehab Waltz. Going home soon now.

Huge advances in after-surgery treatment are being made. One of the more dramatic changes is how the "step down" in care is being made. In many hospitals, the patient stays in the same bed for the duration of the hospital stay. A growing body of evidence demonstrates the effect of this change. The most notable and perhaps the most important of the changes is that the patient isn't required to stay as long.

Another change occurs when the patient must get out of bed to learn the rehab waltz. These two changes have reduced the hospital time by 20 percent or more. These changes have reduced the overall procedure costs and improved the recovery process.

You may have noticed the tone of this has gotten lighter—for good reason. You are making real progress. Besides, your insurance might run out. Well, not really. My cardiologist pointed out that he has never heard of single case of someone being thrown out of the hospital because the insurance ran out. Remember we mentioned nothing would happen until the medical establishment learned how they would be paid. But what is important is the shift of focus to aftercare.

Yes, the real breakthrough toward survival is the immediate aftercare.

Caregiver notes: The subject of aftercare is so important that I will deal with it in greater detail in just a little bit. Suffice it to say for now, the patient will need a lot of TLC for the first six weeks after the surgery, and that TLC has to come from many sources.

Several things will begin to happen that are the real signs the hospital is getting ready to make your bed available for someone else. For instance, the nurses will not be so available to give you pain meds. Nor will they be so tolerant of any little complaints you might have. They are just getting you ready to go home. In con game terms, this is called "The Kiss Off."

Caregiver notes: Your patient may begin to complain about the noticeable decline in level of care. This is your cue. Your patient is on the verge of being released and now your real work is about to begin. In this next section, we will begin to discuss, among other things, patient proofing the living quarters. You will also have to prepare yourself for the onslaught of tasks that you will have to provide. The first several weeks of home care are not much different from caring for a small child; a very large and vocal small child.

One of our vetters has informed us that the time in the CICU is now only one to two days. Further, the scary endotracheal tube may be pulled out by the time the patient wakes up. This is good news for all concerned.

Surgery Aftermath or Getting Your Life Back Together

It comes as somewhat of a shock that you are kicked out of the hospital so soon after surgery. You know you are as good as out when they pull the last of the lines, almost totally ignore you, and give you several pages of instructions to follow when you go home. A nurse or an aide of some kind will bring in a bunch of forms for you to sign attesting to the fact you have received all those pages of instructions. Lastly, an aide will show up with a wheelchair for your last ride in the hospital. That aide will stick around to make sure someone is picking you up and you have no plans to drive yourself home. Don't laugh; there are cases of people thinking they would be able to do just that.

Caregiver notes: It will be incumbent upon you to get the medications list before your patient gets out the door. Make sure you have the total list of the drugs, the schedule of their dispensing, and the correct dosages. Do not rely on the labels to supply all the information. Understand this list and educate your patient. The more ownership you can pass to your patient as to drugs and times of day to take them, the sooner you will have one less thing to worry about.

Be there when the list of instructions is reviewed. Your patient is not going to remember what those instructions are. And the instructions are important.

While in the hospital, all medications are charted and recorded on an official form called a MAR, Medicine Administration Record. The form is a grid that has the times of the day across the top to form columns and the pre-scribed medications down the side to form the rows. When a nurse administers the medicines, a record in made in the appropriate block as to administering nurse and the time given. This is an official part of the patient's chart. It would be a good idea for you to establish such a form for your use.

The next six or seven weeks will seem like a protracted exercise in discomfort. As bad as it is, it is really all downhill from this point on. Consider this: the total estimated time from surgery to the ability to return to work (depending on what you do for a living) is twelve weeks. The administrators down at the old Unemployment Compensation Bureau start to take a dim view if you try to take more time off. Your doctors (both your internist and your cardiologist) will have to write letters of justification. And remember, your doctors survive by knowing what the limits are.

Caregiver notes: Before reading what the patient's first several weeks of life will be like when coming home from surgery, we need to spend some time discussing getting the home ready for the patient. A little preparation on your part can save tons of agony for the patient and aggravation for you. You will need to do a "gap" analysis of what the home looks like now and what will facilitate the patient's recovery.

Some physical considerations include how the patient will get up and down stairs, shower water temperature, toilet usage, and getting in and out of bed and chairs. Things taken for granted will suddenly become major hurdles to overcome. A "little" thing like getting in and out of bed becomes a major undertaking when the patient has great difficultly swinging feet up and down.

A recovering cardiac surgery patient is extremely sensitive to sudden changes in water temperature; water will seem either very hot or very cold. Finding the most acceptable temperature will take some tinkering and you, as caregiver, will have to make sure the temperature is acceptable and tolerable. The sensitivity is the result of anemia. There is just not enough iron in the blood. Even with strong iron supplements, it can take up to six weeks for the red blood cell levels to increase to prevent the sensitivity.

Carefully consider bed height. In our case, our bed is on the high side. My patient could not get his feet up when he first came home. Getting into bed was like mountain climbing. Our son built a step platform to accommodate and facilitate bed entry and exit. You might be able to get by with a single step. Whatever your solution, you must be there to watch and help. You do not want your patient falling.

A good sturdy shower stool or chair will also be required. Do not use anything that could shatter. Our first stool was made of plastic and, although it said it could hold 300 pounds, it could not hold 190 pounds. It shattered, leaving my patient on the shower stall floor, helpless to get up. It was a scary moment. We replaced that stool with a sturdy shower chair purchased from a medical supplies store.

Food preparation will become of paramount importance. Not only will you have to carefully consider what you make, you will have to think about where your patient will eat. Your patient cannot be making many trips up and down the stairs for meals. The patient will have to have some, if not all, meals in bed for some period. You will need to accommodate this requirement in the beginning but you must also begin encouraging the patient to get out of bed and down the steps.

This is the tough part: Your patient is probably used to doing everything for himself. You are used to this being the fact. It all changes. The patient is almost helpless. The patient has no energy so everything is a great effort. The patient is in continual pain and everything is an irritation. The patient cannot prepare food and, worse, has no appetite. As difficult as it is for the patient, it will be likewise difficult for you. When the patient can't sleep, you will not be able to sleep. When the patient naps, you won't be able to nap in case the patient should suddenly awaken and cry out. If you do not think you are up to all this, get help. You will have a sick baby on your hands for a few weeks.

We will soon discuss the effect on you of stress and depression. We mention this early on so it will come as no shock to you when we get into the nitty-gritty. Several of the reviewers and vetters described the adverse effects of depression on the caregivers and how this is a real problem that nobody seems willing or able to address. In particular, Ellen Webb, a nurse; Lorraine Bell, a nurse and caregiver; and Dan Morris, a caregiver, thought we should spend a little more time on this subject. We do just that in the section on stress and depression.

Here is what you can expect the first many weeks home from the hospital:

- Do not try to lift anything heavier than five pounds, no exceptions. Your sternum and your chest muscles cannot possibly survive any greater effort and you will end up back in the emergency room. Plus, the pain will be unbearable.
- A hot shower will be most welcome. Get help taking it. Get a shower stool or chair and relax awhile under the warm water. Wash your hair several times. Shave. Whatever you shave,

shave it. For some reason, making yourself feel clean is uplifting.

- You will feel cold. It will seem no amount of heat will warm you up. Wear warm clothes. You are cold from lack of calories; eating tons of food will not help. Your body is still in shock from the surgery and the cold is a coping mechanism.

- You might be told you have a "food" holiday for a few weeks and you can eat some foods high in fat. Do not take that holiday. It is imperative you get on the new diet, adapt to the new lifestyle, and get completely acclimated to it.

- You will have a follow-up visit with your cardiologist and a complete explanation of all that was done to you. The cardiologist will also give you a prognosis. Here is what you should hear regardless of the words the cardiologist uses: "You will die if you do not get on the regime and stay on it. You are lucky. You dodged the bullet this time. You might not be so lucky the next time."

- The cardiologist will send you to a Cardio Fit rehab program. This is an exercise program that lasts thirty-six sessions and longer depending on your advancement and your insurance limitations.

- Start walking for as long as you can even if it is only pacing around the house. Motion is important for recovery.

- You will be depressed. There is much written about that depression later in this book.

- You will have no appetite. Don't worry about it. Losing weight is best for you in the long run. You will start to eat in a few weeks no matter what else happens. However, the more you can eat of the right foods in the beginning of your recovery period, the quicker your recovery.

- Start taking a good multipurpose vitamin with iron.
- Don't even think about driving yourself anywhere.
- You will have your last follow-up with the surgeon. The surgeon will tell you everything that was done to you. With luck, you will never see the surgeon again. Unfortunately, for me, I did see the surgeon again. I did not see him until the day before the second surgery. When he came into my hospital room, I started the conversation by saying, "Doc, we have to stop meeting this way."
- It is not really necessary, but it is nice if you thank the surgeon for saving your life. You don't have to send flowers. Candy might be nice. Especially butter creams.
- It is also nice to thank the cardiologist for the same thing but you will be seeing the cardiologist for the rest of your life. I don't think the cardiologist will find it funny if you send butter creams.
- Take your drugs as prescribed. Don't mess around with this. You have been given those drugs for a reason. They are not optional. (Refer back to the sections on Measurement and Testing.)
- Make and carry a list of all the drugs you take and the schedule of administration.
  - This is another of those things that seems to get lost in translation as you recover. We carry a card. Banner Boswell gives out pill vials that are easy to open. They even

provide a set of forms to be kept on the vial listing all your medical vitals. We think men prefer the cards (easy to carry in a billfold) and women prefer the vial (just one more thing in the handbag.). This could save your life.

- You will be tired. Naps are important. But do not nap so much during the day that you cannot sleep at night. Sleeplessness at night will cause you to want to take sleep medication. You will want to stop taking that stuff as soon as you can. I learned the trick of lying in bed and keeping perfectly still. There was no stimulus from outside sources. No radio or television blaring away. I would just zone out for an hour at a time. This proved very restful. I can still do this, many years after the surgery.

- Get yourself a Medic Alert[20] bracelet or necklace. This could save your life.

- If you start to feel like you are having a heart attack, get to an emergency room. Dial 911. Don't take any chances. Until my heart was totally repaired, I was a familiar face at my emergency room. I was on a first-name basis with almost the entire staff. They even had my picture in the waiting room. This is the truth.

Caregiver notes: Please learn and understand the above list. The diet part is important and you may want to learn to eat the same foods as your patient. This provides several benefits:

---

20   Medic Alert, 2323 Colorado Ave., Turlock, Ca., 95382. 1 800 432 5378. E-mail: customerservice@medicalert.org

- *You will not have to prepare two different meals.*
- *You will encourage your patient to eat smart.*
- *You will lose weight and lower your cholesterol levels.*
  - *Better than curing heart disease is preventing it.*
- *Eliminate temptation for the patient to cheat.*
- *You can take the attitude of: "If you can eat it I can too."*
- *If you have to eat it, you might take a few extra steps to make the food taste good.*
- *No salt.*
- *No fat.*
- *No fooling.*

Food is essential to recovery. Your patient will need at least fifteen hundred calories a day. Getting that number of proper calories down the gullet of your patient is no easy feat. The drugs are appetite killers, especially the pain meds. Without good nutrition during this phase of recovery, depression is worse. One of the few foods your patient will be able to eat with little complaint is egg. You will need to have Egg Beaters in adequate supply. You may not use whole eggs. You may use egg whites. No yolk is no joke.

Besides having a bad appetite, your patient is going to be cold. Warm pajamas are a must. The patient will be especially cold at night. An extra blanket is necessary. The only thing that is going to reduce the need for extra external warmth is exercise. If you are up to it, and you are going to have to be up to it, get your patient out of bed and walking around the house for five to ten minutes many times a day; the more exercise, the better.

As soon as possible, you want to get the patient out of the house and walking for ten to fifteen minutes. Try to extend the time and length of the walks and rest often. In the beginning, it is perfectly permissible to make your patient walk for five minutes and then stand still for two or three minutes and then walk for another five minutes.

As time goes by, your patient will show better and better recovery. You know a big corner has been turned when your patient wants to go out for dinner. This demonstrates

1. Your patient is taking an interest in things other than the sick heart,
2. Your patient's appetite is returning, and
3. Your patient requires a change of scene.

These are all positive signs.

When the visiting nurse shows up, make sure you cover your patient's exercise schedule. The nurse will also want to cover diet issues and medication adherence. The nurse will take the vitals and will draw blood for the continual testing required in the early days of recovery. Having the nurse draw the blood will mitigate the number of times you have to schlep the patient to the lab.

If your patient has been prescribed a Cardio Fit rehabilitation program, stick around and watch. All the exercise is based on a schedule of exercise for a short period and rest, then exercise again and rest. As improvement is demonstrated, the exercise periods will be lengthened and the rest periods shortened. The aim of the exercise is to build stamina and strength. One-pound weights will be used and the weights will be slowly increased.

In the very beginning of the program, at Level One, the patient will probably wear a monitor transmitting to a nurse's station. The supervising attendant will monitor your patient and stop the exercise if any problem is detected. Many of these programs are performed in a hospital. This is a good idea if an emergency arises. Be prepared, sometimes an emergency does arise. As a caregiver, I attended *all those early sessions. On more than one occasion, it was necessary to get my patient to the ER. It was comforting to know help was only moments away.*

The Cardio Fit people keep an exercise log. The log is sent to the cardiologist to review. You may want to establish such a log for your patient. This log is to record exercise outside of Cardio Fit. It will be a good thing to show both the cardiologist and the visiting nurse.

The supervising attendant will take blood pressure and pulse several times during the exercise period. Everything the patient does is recorded and that information is forwarded to the cardiologist. You will see the doctors often in the first three months after surgery.

The cardiologist monitors heart recovery and the entire range of issues attendant to that recovery. Your internist, on the other hand, monitors everything else. There are many things that must be monitored, especially drug levels in the blood. If brand name Coumadin (warfarin) or other generic blood thinner is being used, the International Normalized Ratio (INR), or thinness level of the blood, must be continually checked. The way the cardiologist and internist practices are established will determine which doctor will perform which services. You will have a lifetime of adherence to the rules. Get used to them early.

All of the above really fall into the category of aftercare. However, not included in the above is the requirement for emotional support. As important as the physical requirements of the aftercare are, the emotional requirements may be more important.

After surgery, your patient is going to feel isolated. The patient will have limited allowed mobility (no nightclubbing, dancing, and wild parties) and will spend most of the time in bed. The drugs will make reading and television watching difficult, as the drugs prevent the ability to really concentrate. Even long conversations will be difficult.

These things make family and friends very important. Frequent short visits from those near and dear make the days shorter and the burden for both patient and caregiver lighter. However, as the caregiver, you must exercise some discipline as to visit times, refreshments, and duration. You must make visitors understand, as tactfully as possible, that the patient is capable of just so much and no more.

In our case, we were fortunate to have one of our sons with us, plus my patient's mom, my patient's favorite uncle, and some first cousins were all nearby. These folks made regular visits. We also had some friends in the immediate area and they likewise dropped by.

There is something comforting to the patient about being in a familiar place with familiar people and things, including pets, nearby. These things alleviate the feeling of isolation.

Lastly on this subject, you are going to need to be given an occasional break from all your duties. It is nice to have family and friends to fall back on for support. More importantly, the patient will feel safe and comfortable when you are not available. Toward the end of the book, we will be discussing the mental strain heart disease places on you and the patient. The few things I have mentioned here will be much more important when we have that discussion.

Moving Up and Moving On

If you have assiduously followed the instructions above, and you have managed to get your lame butt through those first six or seven weeks, you should face the east and give thanks to the powers that be. Now all you have to learn how to do is to live with the disease and still lead an active and happy life. To paraphrase Macbeth: "Read on, Macduff."[21]

Caregiver notes: The worst is over. You may now have your nervous breakdown.

౿

---

21 **Macduff** is a fictional character in Shakespeare's *Macbeth* (c.1603–1607). He suspects Macbeth of regicide and kills him offstage in the final act.

SECTION TWO –
LIVING WITH CORONARY
ARTERY DISEASE

Setting out to define how to live with CAD is fraught with problems. CAD is not a "one size fits all" proposition. Not every patient fits the exact same profile. CAD comes in a variety of disease manifestations and every patient can react to the disease in a unique manner. CAD patients may have other medical complications, like diabetes or pulmonary disease. Other medical complications constrain the holistic view of the patient's care.

I can't address all that stuff. I am not a doctor and even if I were, I would neither suppose nor propose I could fix all with a magic potion. I am going for the majority of the folks with CAD. As such, there will be some exceptions to the rules. If you read a section and say to yourself, "That isn't me," that is all right. If I am writing about being over-weight, and you are thin, as Steve Martin[22] would say, "Well excuuuuse me." You get the idea. If it is not you, then it is not you, but it probably is about the one sitting next to you.

Think of living with CAD as sitting on a three-legged stool. As long as you have all three legs intact and the same length, sitting can be fairly comfortable. But, shorten any of the legs or ignore or break any of the three legs, and sitting becomes rather precarious, if not just down-right deadly. When I was first diagnosed with CAD, my new friend, the cardiologist, did not mince any words with me. This proved to be an invaluable approach. Cut to the chase and let the chips fall where they may. Mixed metaphors are a pain in the butt and so is living with CAD.

While this book was being reviewed, some of the review-ers expressed a concern that I was not very politically cor-rect. The reviewers thought I was too direct and I might hurt some feelings and turn off some readers. I am not going

22 **Stephen Glenn "Steve" Martin** (born August 14, 1945) is an American actor, comedian, writer, playwright, producer, musician, and composer

to mince words. I am not going to say, "Please stop this or please do this or would you be so kind as to accommodate this change." Your doctor and his or her staff use that language. I can see with my own eyes how far this has gotten them. And the statistics, as stated in just a few pages, back up my observations.

The idea of not mincing words is a philosophical construct or concept. This is important only insofar as I have had to change my life to conform to a set of philosophical tenets. Here are those tenets, some of which I will explain now and the rest will become apparent as you read the rest of the book.

Philosophical Tenets

Tenet One: Acknowledge the situation for what it really is. Before you can really start to get better for the long term, you must **acknowledge** how you got to where you are. In a commercial for one of the many cholesterol drugs, John, age fifty-eight, asks, "What was I thinking about?" Good question. It is too late to feel guilty about all the sins of your past, but it is necessary to acknowledge what you have been doing that is harmful. I have had to acknowledge how I got sick (a most painful evaluation of my health life). If you don't acknowledge the truth of it all, you can't move on.

In an earlier section I wrote about I how got to the surgeon. I acknowledged how I got to my current condition and understood just how stupid I had been. Then I was able to start getting better.

Tenet Two: Accept ownership. This is your problem. Do not try to get someone else to be responsible for the problem, and this especially includes your family and your doctor.

Tenet Three: Agree on what has to be done to move on.
You need to get educated and you need to understand
the what and the why of your treatment. Reading this book
is a big step in the right direction.

Tenet Four: Commit to making the changes. If you are not
willing to make the changes and stick to those changes,
do nothing.

Tenet Five: Change your life. Your CAD diagnosis has al-
tered the journey of your life. If you really want to move on,
you are going to have to make some substantial changes.
We are going to address them all.

Tenet Six: Prepare for the future. CAD has aroused the
need to fight harder if you are to maintain and survive.
CAD is, truthfully, a pronouncement of your mortality. It
is not a death sentence. It is a quest for health that you
did not have prior to the diagnosis. The idea is to die from
something else before the disease eventually reaches the
end state.

Living with CAD is both a metaphysical and a physical journey. It is metaphysical in the need to completely
change your attitude about virtually everything, and
physical in the actual living and doing of the appropriate
lifestyle.

Before getting to the three-legged stool, it is necessary
to set out some rules of acceptance.

Rules of Acceptance

First rule of acceptance: If you are suffering with CAD or
any other long-term cardiac problem, the chances are it
is entirely your fault. Oh, sure, the makers of Vytorin (one of

the many drugs that have come under strict FDA review because of the company's claims and proven efficacy)[23] and the other cardiac drugs advertise that the problem can come from your relatives and is genetic in nature; however, that does not absolve you of living with the problem. You must come to grips with this and **accept the problem as your own**. Blaming your Uncle Irving, Aunt Wanda and your parents is not going to make it any easier.

Your genes load the atherosclerosis gun…but your environment of poor diet, lack of exercise, stress, and anxiety is what pulls the trigger[24].

Caregiver notes: Not only is it hard for the patient to accept the terms and conditions of living, the caregiver must also come to grips with "who owns the disease." It will be necessary to remind your patient who has the ultimate responsibility for the disease. Here is a clue—it is not the caregiver. Under no circumstances should a caregiver assume any of the responsibility for the disease. A caregiver is there to support, tend to, and, if possible, give love and tender mercy to the patient. The caregiver does not take the medicine. **Second rule of acceptance**: You are too damn fat. I tried to kill myself with my knife, fork, and spoon (not to mention the forests worth of chopsticks) for many years. I was fifty pounds overweight. I deluded myself into thinking that it was all right to be "just moderately" overweight. Baloney. For every fat pound you carry around, your body has to produce a mile of arteries and veins and your heart has to

---

23   Dr. Greg Quinn, cardiologist, pointed out: The study comparing the effects of Simvastatin vs Vytorin revealed no significant difference in carotid intimal thickness within a unique population that is not truly representative of the majority with CAD. Much was made of insignificant trends suggesting a detrimental effect of Vytorin. Many have speculated much of the debate and negative press reflects efforts by competing entities to increase market share.

24   Dr. Steven Raskin, Cardiologist, Alameda, California

get the blood through all that mass of ice cream, butter, and salty junk food. In body physiology terms, it is twice as hard for the heart to pump blood through all that junk as to pump blood through muscle.

Being overly gifted in the big belly causes serious physical restrictions on your ability to breathe. Your heart, already taxed by disease, must contend with lungs that have nowhere to go to expand and get oxygen to your muscles. The mechanical reasons for this will be discussed in the section on Heart Disease and Chronic Obstructive Pulmonary Disease.

Remember this: Fast food is fat food. Unlike an apple, a burger a day will kill you. If you are more than fifty pounds overweight, you are, by definition, obese.[25] **Accept this fact, and then start to change it.**

Caregiver notes: We all have a tendency to "pork up" over years of life together. No fault is being laid on here—merely an observation. Our hectic schedules have caused us to create shortcuts and one of those shortcuts is fast or convenience foods and dining out. All of these shortcuts now belong to the no-no list. The extra poundage put on over the past many years will now have to come off. This is no longer just to look better. In the patient's case, it could be a matter of life or death.

---

25 From WebMD. Obesity is an excess proportion of total body fat. A person is considered obese when his or her weight is 20 percent or more above normal weight. The most common measure of obesity is the body mass index or BMI. A person is considered overweight if his or her BMI is between 25 and 29.9; a person is considered obese if his or her BMI is over 30. "Morbid obesity" means that a person is either 50 percent to 100 percent over normal weight, more than one hundred pounds over normal weight, has a BMI of 40 or higher, or is sufficiently overweight to severely interfere with health or normal function.

Third rule of acceptance: If you smoke, you are a moron.[26] Not only that, but if you smoke, you are not only a moron, you stink. And if you are still smoking after having a heart attack and being diagnosed with CAD or other serious heart disease, please stop going to see your doctor. He or she has better things to do than try to keep you alive while you are doing so much damage to yourself. Get out of the way so the doctor has time to spend with people who are actually trying to get better. Besides, your stupidity is costing me, as an American taxpayer, real money to keep you alive. And I have no desire to enrich the tobacco industry secondhand. Also, secondhand smoke does kill. And you still stink.

(Lee Iacocca[27], while he was running Chrysler said, "Employees came in three styles. They either led, followed, or were in the way." Lee is probably not the first to say this. If you smoke, you are in the way.)

Here is more good news about smoking. Smoking as few as ten cigarettes a day places the same strain on the cardiovascular systems as carrying around an extra fifty pounds. Wow, how good for you, the smoker. You don't have to eat too much to enjoy the benefits of being obese. The tobacco companies are making obesity unnecessary. At only $6 a pack you too can receive the same benefit of eating six value-priced hamburgers. What a good deal that is.

---

26 Dictionary.com definition
1. A person who is notably stupid or lacking in good judgment.
2. *Psychology.* A person of borderline intelligence in a former classification of mental retardation, having an intelligence quotient of 50 to 69. Now considered offensive.

27 **Lido Anthony "Lee" Iacocca** (born October 15, 1924) is an American businessman known for his revival of the Chrysler Corporation in the 1980s, serving as President and CEO from 1978 and additionally as chairman from 1979, until his retirement at the end of 1992. One of the most famous business people in the world, he was a passionate advocate of U.S.

Caregiver notes: Cough, cough, pee yew, stink, stink. You smell so bad you make me blink.

Fourth rule of acceptance: The changes you must make are for the rest of your life. Most people, approximately 50 percent, unfortunately, revert to all their old bad habits within a mere two years of being diagnosed. By the third year, 50 percent of the remaining 50 percent fall off the wagon. By the fourth year, another 50 percent resume the bad old ways. And by the seventh year, only 3–4 percent have made the true conversion required to stay alive.[28] The result of the backsliding: back to the emergency room. Worst result: the reoccurrence kills them. I say goody. More care for me. And others like me who are actually trying to stay well.

Caregiver notes: These are the statistics referred to in the preface and just a few pages ago. In a mere two years, 50 percent throw in the towel and resume all the bad old habits abandoned when first diagnosed. The reasons given are usually lame excuses like too hard to stay on the diet, travel makes it too hard, no support at home, my favorite team is in last place, etc. Your job, as the caregiver, is to make sure there is no backsliding. The options are not pretty.

Earlier, in the section about Open Heart Surgery, I mentioned the need for options. I made that comment because of an experience we had pertaining the writing of this book. We solicited the help of many people in the writing. Many we solicited help from are cardiac patients. (For those that helped and were generous with their comments and encouragement, let me give a big shout-out of thanks.)

---

28 I found these statistics in several places, including WebMD and the American Heart Association. WebMD referenced the Cleveland Heart Clinic, which, by the way, is rated as the best Cardiac Hospital in America. But hey, that's what *U.S. News and World Report* had to say in their August 2009 edition and who am I to argue?

We approached a man who was starting his third round of cardio rehab after having his third open-heart surgery. Yes, Virginia, this man is Santa Claus to some cardio surgeon. The man was morbidly obese, weighing in the three hundred pound plus range. We asked if he would read the book and give us his input. He refused, saying this was his third round of rehab and he knew all about it. We wondered what he knows all about. He has had three open-heart surgeries, and he is more than one hundred pounds overweight.

Fifth rule of acceptance: You are not alone. Others have already been this way before. You are not the last of the Mohicans or the first pioneer to travel this path. You are depressed and unhappy and believe that no one can understand what you are going through. More baloney. No matter how sick you think you are now, many others have been much sicker and now live comfortably. So get over yourself. If you ever meet me, please don't try to tell me how bad you have had it. Been there, done that, have the T-shirt, coffee mug, heart-shaped pillow, and scars to prove it. I won't tell you how bad I had it either.

Caregiver notes: Your patient is going to be a real pain in the butt by feeling sorry for him or herself. Your patient will believe "nobody knows the trouble I seen," to quote the spiritual. You must disabuse the patient of this silly idea. Ridicule might work, but I don't recommend it. Then again, ridicule might be the only thing that will work.

Sixth rule of acceptance: You need someone to talk to about what you are going through. You will be self-obsessed (remember the man with the golden screw in his belly button?) with your sickness and the depression that almost always accompanies any kind of heart procedure will make you feel your heart weighs a million pounds.

You will also be wary of even the slightest chest pain and will think nothing of showing up at the emergency room screaming, "Heart attack, heart attack!" If you have had open-heart surgery, you are going to be very stressed and very depressed. I'll have much more to say about that in just a skosh. (I have no idea why it is called "open-heart surgery." Most heart procedures are bypass surgery and your heart is not opened up. Your heart is opened up if they are replacing failed valves. I think it should be called "open-chest surgery.")

Caregiver notes: Your patient is going to be doing a lot of complaining and will feel the continual need to "unburden" the pain and grief. You are going to have to grin and bear it. However, you are going to need someone to talk to and it can't be the patient. You will need a friend to confide in. For reasons not understood, the medical community does something less than an adequate job in looking after the health of the caregiver. But then, why should they? After all, in our experience, caregiver stress syndrome is not a recognized condition. I don't know of any support groups. We have been told such things might exist in other communities and towns, just not here. You will have to ask your cardiologist or internist where you live. Who would have time to attend? Being a full-time caregiver is a full-double-time job.

Seventh rule of acceptance: <u>Follow all the directions</u> you receive from your health care professionals. You can't say to yourself, "I like this direction, but I don't like this other one, so I'll forget about it." To this I say, "Here is what you can do with that attitude." I make an obscene gesture while I am saying this. Of course, I do smile all the while.

Caregiver notes: Have you ever met a patient that follows all the directions? Neither have I. However, there can be no shirking the directions.

Eighth rule of acceptance: Take it all personally. Take all that I am writing here as a personal attack. Think about what is being said. This is all in-your-face stuff we are discussing. If you don't take it personally, I am wasting my time and yours. Go watch some cartoons. Or read the latest edition of the *National Enquirer*. Both are probably more on your intelligence level.

Caregiver notes: If your patient doesn't take it personally, you should. This is a lifetime commitment.

Ninth rule of acceptance: Get educated. Coronary disease is both a silent and a passive disease. And it stays both silent and passive until the artery wall ruptures or a block occurs. It affects the most important muscle in your body and, by definition, anything that can go wrong, will go wrong. The heart walls have thinned and this most important pump is straining to do its work. Education leads to you to think, thought leads to enlightenment, and enlightenment leads to positive action. Not only will you understand what is wrong and why, you will be motivated to take care of yourself. At least that's the plan. You have no idea how much literature there is that is easily available and free. You can always ask your cardiologist or primary care doctor. The only stupid question, in this case, is the unasked and unanswered one.

Caregiver notes: We are all unprepared when the first serious cardiac event occurs. By reading this, you are taking a big step forward in understanding what is going on and why. Getting educated and informed is a "dirty job" but somebody has to do it. Otherwise, you will flounder around in dread, desperation, and despair.

Dread, desperation, and despair lead to extra amounts of stress on you, as if you need anymore. This stress is very wearing, and it will literally grind you down. You will become depressed yourself and now there are two depressed people instead of only one.

Heart patients can suffer from an under diagnosed disease called SAD. SAD means Stressed, Anxious, and Depressed. (This may get confusing for some. SAD stands for Seasonal Affective Disorder. It's a type of depression that is very well known in the medical community and even in the lay press.[29]) It is usually not communicable. Being a non-communicable disease does not mean you cannot catch it. Be wary. There will be much discussion about this later.

Tenth rule of acceptance: You are going to need a support network to help you heal. You cannot get through this alone. I was very fortunate. My wife saw what I was going through, understood at an emotional level what my needs were going to be, and was there to help me. And in all honesty, I must admit there were some very dark days ahead for me and for her. It is also why she coauthored this book.

Eleventh rule of acceptance: The path to recovery is almost identical to the path traveled by someone coping with the loss of a loved one. An important part of your life will be taken away from you and you will have to grieve for that loss. Your id, ego, and libido are all going to take big hits. Not acknowledging these hits will multiply your stress and depression levels. Since stress and depression are negative in nature, on a scale of 1 to 10 you will probably feel like a −18.

---

29 Dr. Mark Moeller, M.D. Family Practice, Sutter West Medical Group, Davis, Ca.

Caregiver notes: We will spend quite a bit of time discussing the issue of depression a little later in the book. Nobody tells you about this issue, and the docs do a rotten job of acknowledging and treating the problem. In retrospect, we found this rather astounding. My patient was greatly depressed after both operations. The prescribed treatment was drugs. This is a case of that good old American fall-back position of not addressing the problem head-on but instead relying on pharmaceuticals to treat the symptoms. In many cases this approach is both bad and dangerous. Your patient is going to be depressed and you must get prepared for it. (In the right situation psych medications are as or more important than diuretics or beta blockers. The right antidepressant medications in the right individuals can save lives.[30])

A Parable for Our Times

A bird got a late start in flying south at the changing of the seasons. The bird ran right into a heavy sleet storm and was driven to the ground by the cold and the weight of the precipitation. He lay freezing on the ground and thought to himself, "It can't get any worse, I am doomed to die."

What the bird did not know was he had landed in a farm. A short while later a big cow passed over the bird and did what cows are wont to do and dropped a large cow patty right on the bird. "Oh great!" the bird thought. "It can't get any worse than this. I am doomed to die in a heap of cow plop." But a funny thing happened. The cow plop was warm and quickly thawed the bird. The bird then did what birds are wont to do and he stuck his head out of the cow plop and started to sing.

The barn cat heard this strange thing, a singing cow patty, and went to investigate, being curious, as cats are

30 Dr. Mark Moeller, M.D. Family Practice, Sutter West Medical Group, Davis, Ca

wont to be. The cat pawed through the plop, found the bird, and ate it. Too bad, so sad.

In this story, the bird was just being a bird, the cow was just being a cow, and the cat was just being a cat. Nothing good or bad is either explicit or implicit in the story. No judgments are being made. The lessons of the story are these:

1. When it is time to get out of town, get out of town. Don't hang around thinking things are going to get better. Things never get better, they only get worse. This is in keeping with a principal law of physics: all things left to themselves tend to decay into chaos.

2. All those who put you in a plop are not necessarily your enemies.

3. All those who pull you out of a plop are not necessarily your friends.

4. And most of important of all—If you should find yourself in a plop and are warm and happy, keep your mouth shut.

The Three-Legged Stool

The three legs of the stool are **diet, exercise, and medications**, listed in no particular order of importance. All are equally important. One other thing is also very important. It is helpful if your cardiologist appears to care about you, not just as a patient, but also as a person. An unusual trait of the doctor is the annoying circumstance of the doctor always running late. The biggest contributor to the running late syndrome is the doctor is taking the time to explain, in detail, what is going on with somebody's heart. Remember, the doc will take time with you too.

I have observed that cardiologists are generally overworked and, in my opinion, under compensated. "How can this be?" you ask. You need to know how the insurance companies pay claims. It is an arcane system that is used by private insurers and Medicare. Doctors are paid for a unit of work, called RVU's ((relative value units)), which involves a complex and completely illogical collection of factors involving difficulty of the decision making, time spent, procedures done, etc.

In the U.S., doctors are not paid for how much time they spend with patients or for how much their care and work benefits the patients. That is an important point; doctors get paid for how much they do but not for how well they do it. They are paid by the RVU, which tend to be much greater for the number of drugs prescribed and significantly greater for running tests and procedures.

Most doctors are very well intentioned and try to ignore the RVU's and simply do what's best for their patients, but given how much more doctors make for running tests and doing procedures you stay vigilant about asking why and what for. The RVU's are proscribed by law (Medicare) or policy (private insurers which, among other things, has time limitations placed on that unit of work and is called, in insurance parlance, a level of service.

The time limits are dictated by law (Medicare) or policy (private insurers). The doctor has only so much time per patient, and if he or she runs over that time, the doctor is paying for that time out of his or her own pocket. So if the doctor is late, he or she is paying for it personally. That is one definition of dedicated.

Another controlling factor in the use of the doctors' time is the insurance company policy of "capitation." The insurance companies, particularly the health plans, invented capitation as a way to control the costs of health care. With capitation, a person is no longer a person but a "life" (cool, huh?). All the participating doctors subscribing to the insurance health plan automatically receive a monthly check to ensure delivery of service. This is meant to motivate doctors to keep patients healthy because healthy patients are far less expensive to a capitated system than sick patients but it doesn't always work that way.

Caregiver notes: There is an exemption and exception to this rule. Some docs are so busy they do not take the time to cover everything that should be covered. It is your job as caregiver to say, "Hold up there, Bucko, explain all of this to us." Take nothing for granted and challenge anything and everything the doc tells you. It is the doc's job to keep you informed. You cannot be concerned about the doc's use of time, and how the insurance companies and health plans are controlling the doc.

I feel compelled to issue a warning. If you do not see the doc taking the time to thoroughly examine the chart or medical notes, call a halt to the proceedings. Believe it or not, some docs are so rushed they just start an exam without first reading the pathology. We lived through just such an experience and it led to some very unwelcome circumstances.

It was strongly suggested we tell why we make this warning. Two years ago or so, my husband suddenly started to feel very poorly. The sudden decline in his ability to exercise came for no apparent reason and was both troubling and scary. He was not informed of a change made without his knowledge to his pacer setting. The change to his pacer was made in December and his troubles became very noticeable by the end of that month.

He was scheduled to see his cardiologist the first week of February. He decided to live with it until his scheduled appointment. His health grew gradually worse. Just prior to his appointment, he received a call from the doctor's office wanting to know if he would be willing to see the assistant. No, he wanted to see his doctor. The appointment was rescheduled for two weeks later.

Meanwhile, our anxiety levels were greatly escalating. The symptoms were identical to those he suffered in late 2001. The tests he had in 2001 revealed he had a leak in his heart and his mitral valve was failing. The repair of the leak and the replacement of the mitral valve required a second open-heart surgery, which was done in January of 2002. You can appreciate his fear when he suddenly developed those same bad old symptoms.

Finally he got to see the doctor. The doctor asked how he was doing and my patient told him. Without even reviewing his chart, the doctor started to schedule a full range of tests—all of them time consuming, expensive and aggravating but absolutely necessary.

After all the tests came back negative, I convinced my patient to mention the pacer examination to the doctor. A quick check of the pacer settings revealed the pacer technician had turned off one of the two leads to the heart. The lead was turned back on and, voila, my patient was fine.

If the doctor had taken just a few minutes to read the chart and see the notes from the pacer tech, all the testing would have been avoided. That means all the pain, fear, and aggravation, and the extra out-of-pocket costs would have been eliminated. We now have another cardiologist who reads the notes. This is very important.

I have had several sets of doctors in the past eight years. I have had a chance to evaluate all of them and I have reached several conclusions as to what constitutes good care and what is something less then desirable. Care can be expressed on two levels. The first level is considered "infrastructure" support. The other level, which is where the tire hits the sky, so to speak, is the hands-on delivery of service. The expression, "tire hits the sky", I first heard spoken by a business associate. He was explaining just how difficult it was to deliver good quality.

Infrastructure deals with all the support services required to look after you. This includes everything from greeting you when you enter the office to bookkeeping. The more integrated all of these services are, the easier it is for you. The more use of the new technologies and the adequate training of the folks using the technology, the better it is for you. Is there anyone anymore who doesn't know how to type and use a computer? There may be but I think they live in Third World countries with no electricity or telephones.

The technologies in use today provide the basic recipe for good records. The records are permanent, unchangeable, accurate, and legible. The records stored on these technologies are also secure to comply with HIPAA[31] legislation ensuring privacy. The privacy issues have become so important it is now necessary to stand well back from a person in line for almost any medical transaction. Even a transaction as simple as picking up a prescription or signing in to see the doctor falls under the HIPAA guidelines. You may have noticed the signs that state: "Stand behind this

31   The Health Insurance Portability and Accountability Act of 1996 (HIPAA), Public Law 104–191, was enacted on August 21, 1996. Sections 261 through 264 of HIPAA require the secretary of HHS to publicize standards for the electronic exchange, privacy, and security of health information.

line until it is your turn!" (I wonder if I could get a job as "line cop." Do you think donuts come free as a perk of that job?)

Infrastructure also includes how the offices are laid out and how much room is allocated for each of the medical and business functions. Cramped quarters are a sign of unplanned growth or lack of foresight in laying out the office. Neither is a good sign. Easy access to the business office functions is also undesirable.

Size of the practice has a lot to do with the quality of the infrastructure. A large practice, one with many doctors and services can afford to invest in the technology. In fact, it is poor business practice not to make such investments. Small practices find themselves between a rock and hard place. A small practice must, by necessity, resort to almost everything being done by hand. This results in mistakes, which are expensive and aggravating. Worse, they can cause a serious mistake in your care.

With many doctors looking after your well-being, it is imperative they all share the same medical records. It is time consuming, expensive, stressful, and aggravating to answer the same questions every time you see a doctor. It is worse if you go to a specialist outside the immediate practice and find yourself filling out the forms for insurance, advanced directive, personal medical history, and family medical history (how many times do I have to check off my grandfather had a heart attack?). What is even worse, after you fill out all that history stuff, the doctor never seems to have read it. Comedian Lewis Black[32] has an expression that fits this situation. So did George Carlin[33] and you see where it got him! Unfortunately, I can't repeat it here. You

---

32 **Lewis Niles Black** (born August 30, 1948) is a Grammy Award-winning American stand-up comedian, author, playwright, and actor. He is known for his comedy style, which often includes simulating a mental breakdown or an increasingly angry rant, ridiculing history, politics, religion, trends, and cultural phenomena.

33 **George** Denis Patrick **Carlin** (May 12, 1937 – June 22, 2008) was an American stand-up comedian. He was also an actor and author.

know how these guys talk. You can probably figure it out yourself.

The need to share your medical information becomes even more imperative if the doctor provides many services. In my case, which is not unique, my cardiologist is responsible for not only the ongoing maintenance of my CHF, but for the regular Coumadin testing, the follow-up of exercise regimens, and the diet compliance. Regular blood testing for a variety of things is also part of the service. This cardiologist has not only invested in infrastructure support, he has made big capital investments in all the advanced testing equipment essential to cardiac care. His practice provides more or less one-stop shopping for all my cardiac needs.

The practice's systems provide for the complete sharing of my medical history with the individuals I meet in the delivery of health services. The water gets a little murkier when I have to see other doctors outside of the cardiologist's practice. In some cases, the sharing of the records must be done the old-fashioned way, on paper. In my cardiologist's office, everyone sees and updates the same records (the patient chart).

I also see an internist on a semi-regular basis. I take relatively good care of myself so I don't spend much time with my internist these days. My visits to him are confined to a semi-annual general checkup and the yearly physical. If I am sick, either I go to the ER, if I think it is something serious and related to my heart, or to the urgent care facility that is part of the local health network I belong to as part of my Medicare-paid-for insurance. Lucky me!

I am being very serious about how lucky I am to have this care available. Many do not. In fact, almost 50 million Americans do not have health insurance, which is a large part of why health care is so expensive for those of us who do. We indirectly subsidize all those who don't have insurance and we do so at an enormous premium because the uninsured, ironically, only get the most expensive care (emergency care) and not the least expensive, most important care (preventative care). This is another reason why everything cost so much and you get what you pay for, or in the case of the non-insured, the best of everything that they cannot afford to pay for.

The major benefit of this health care delivery system is the sharing of all medical and financial records. All the docs in the system have access to my insurance information, which cuts way down on all the paperwork. I do have to pay my co-pays at the time of delivery of service, but hey, I don't have to deal with monthly statements. Neither do they. This cuts down costs—the costs of administration—which are eating us all alive.

When our president gives his "State of the Union" address every January, he invariably makes a statement about how technology can cut down the costs of medical care. The technology he is referencing is as much administrative as it is medical. The next time you complain about the cost of medicine, look around your doctor's office and see what is being done to reduce the actual costs associated with being in business.

President Obama[34] has made health care one of his key initiatives. In all of the discussions surrounding the issue of health care, invariably one of the most important, if not the most important, imperatives is the electronic sharing of medical records. The issue of electronic sharing of records is so important President Obama has put a five-year mandate on completing this task. This is no mean feat, as it will require massive reorganization of work procedures and realignment of human resources. The up-front costs to accomplish this initiative will run into the billions of dollars.

---

34 **Barack Hussein Obama II** (born August 4, 1961) is the forty-fourth and current president of the United States. The first African American to hold the office, he served as the junior United States senator from Illinois from January 2005 until he resigned after his election to the presidency in November 2008.

However, this is the fastest and surest way to reduce health care costs for the total population.

Of course, all this comes to naught if the technology is not properly used. This addresses the next area of concern, the quality of care provided by the doctor and the care delivery personnel. I'll bet you think you have the best doctor in the whole world. You don't? Why not?

Good Doctor, Good Patient

There is no such thing as the "best" doctor in the whole world. It is impossible to be the best at anything that is so subjective in nature. What are the characteristics that constitute being the best doctor and how do you measure them? I am not capable of evaluating every doctor. First of all, I can't allow them all to treat me. My first cousin, a doctor, by the by, laughs when he hears someone is considered as the best doctor. He has a standard question, "Who says?" My cousin is very big on challenging assumptions. Challenging assumptions is a good thing.

What are the characteristics that constitute being a "good" doctor? A good doctor implies the nature of the relationship between doctor and patient. A good doctor, in the eyes of the patient, satisfactorily performs the job of doctoring. This would further imply the patient satisfactorily performs the job of being a patient. What is good for the goose is good for the gander.

All things can be measured on a "bell curve." On this curve, 20 percent will fall at the bottom of the curve, 20 percent at the top of the curve, and the remaining 60 percent fall somewhere in the middle. The problem with the bell curve is what do you measure?

When you went to school, it was helpful if you knew how the teacher was grading you. If the teacher was grading on a scale to one hundred, you intrinsically knew what differentiated a bad grade from a good grade. Getting a hundred on a test or assignment assured you a high-class standing. High-class standings were very important. On this scale, grades spoke for themselves. With the scale, you did not worry about the other students. You worried only about what you had to learn. The issue is very cloudy on a curve.

On a curve, you were not graded on how well you learned the subject, but how well you learned it relative to the other students in your class or section. In this instance, the emphasis was on how well you competed. This is OK if you are running a race. It might not be so good if you have to learn how to cut open a human being. (My doctor is best because he can cut open a person better than your doctor. He might have a small problem once the patient is cut open, but he can cut open the person real good.)

In the latter part of the last century, thanks to those that advocated not making people accountable for themselves, a pass/fail system was instituted. This system put no emphasis on how well a student performed and relied on the grader to establish if the student learned "enough." This system always mystified me. I was never able to learn what "enough" was. In the practice of medicine, what is "enough"?

The best that is possible is to evaluate a doctor relative to the perceived value of the care being delivered. It is not "enough" to measure on one aspect of care delivery. Pass/fail could be equated to live/die when it comes to serious cardiac care. All cardiac care is serious.

Education is important in medicine. I have no idea what makes one medical school better than another. However, I am more impressed when a doctor is an alumnus from say Harvard Medical than from say Guadalajara College. No, Harvard cannot possibly train all the doctors needed, and there are many fine medical schools. Some are just finer than others.

To be factual, when it comes to most medical schools there is probably little difference in the quality of the education. One school might have a much more impressive name than another, but the overall quality of the education is still very similar. What is probably far more important is the quality of the residency program the doctor went through. I have no way to evaluate that.

It is also nice to know if the doctor bothered with board certification in his or her specialty. Once a person graduates from medical school, that person is legally a doctor. A doctor may practice any specialty desired with no further education. Board certification is an effort by the medical profession to "weed" out those who might be a disgrace to the profession. We all know nobody has ever been a disgrace to medicine, don't we?

On a personal level, how does your doc communicate with you? If your doctor is terse, appears hesitant to share information, and is distant and cold to you, then you might be better off with somebody else. We all have different communication skill levels and, certainly, we all have different personalities. It is just nice if the doc seems to care about you as a person and is interested in more than just what your complaint of the day might be.

In thinking about what appears on the past few pages, we might be able to make up our own test to evaluate how good our doctor is. Here are the evaluation criteria (and scoring is on a bell curve):

Infrastructure

- Patient records are electronic and are secure, permanent, accurate, legible, and unchangeable.
- Business systems are integrated from check-in through to checkout and scheduling.

- Co-payments are handled at the time of either check-in or checkout and billing systems are effective and efficient.
- Waiting room is neat with comfortable chairs. There is adequate space between chairs, preventing the feeling of being crowded. Recent reading material is provided.
- Toilet facilities are convenient and well maintained.
- Support personnel are friendly, well trained, and efficient. Support personnel are also neatly dressed and presentable in total appearance.
- Practice handles all insurance filings.
- Business offices are secure and non-observable.
- Care facilities (examination rooms, testing rooms, etc.) are neat, uncluttered, and adequate for the number of people and amount of equipment using the space.
- Work areas are free of clutter.
- Wait times for scheduled appointments are less than fifteen minutes. If wait times are going to be longer, you are informed on checking in.
- Support personnel have good telephone manners.
- People flow in the office space is smooth.
- Good use of business technology is employed.
- Investments have been made in upgrading of facilities and training of support staff.
- Investments have been made in current and appropriate technology.

Care Delivery

- Professional staff are all properly certified.

- Doctor has graduated from a respected medical school.
- Doctor is board certified.
- Doctor and staff understand and use appropriate medical technology.
- Doctor takes time to understand your problems and concerns.
- Doctor demonstrates some level of empathy and sympathy.
- Doctor takes time to review your medical records and is familiar with your history and pathology.
- Doctor understands your personal history and current situation.

Other things make up what you might consider a "good" doctor. It is necessary to feel comfortable with your doctor. Personal biases are hard to discuss and can shade our thinking without benefit of facts. It is necessary to put aside those biases. The best doctor for you might not be one that comes from your part of the country, has your skin color, is the gender you prefer, practices your religion, or shares your political views.

Doctors and patients alike share some common responsibilities. If you expect the doctor to care about you, you must care about the doctor. This means you must go to the doctor prepared for the visit. The doctor does not have time to play guessing games with you about what is ailing you. There are some things you must always have with you when you go for the visit:

- Your current medicine list (but then you should always have this on your person).
- A list of anything that has changed since your last visit.

- A list of the items you wish to discuss with the doctor including questions about your current course of treatment.
- Be prepared to give the doctor a quick recap of all the things you are doing to comply with the agreed upon treatment plan including your exercise, diet, and medicines.
- A reminder about the other doctors you are seeing and what regimes they have you on.
- The courage to speak up when you feel you are not getting proper care.

Caregiver notes: Many folks hold doctors in some degree of awe and do not challenge anything they say. This is not a good practice. It is incumbent on you as a caregiver not to let anything go by. It is also incumbent on you to ensure your patient has the items listed. You are still the team captain, regardless of however long the treatment has been ongoing.

The welfare of your patient and loved one is at stake so it is very hard to be objective. One way of attaining a true state of objectivity is to reposition the playing field. You are not a supplicant, neither is your patient. The doctor has been "hired" and the doctor's job is to help ensure the patient's ongoing good health. If a plumber comes into your home, you would not hesitate to make sure you understand what the plumber has done and why. What is different? Oh, right, the doctor went to school for a trillion years, charges more per hour, and does not come to your home.

Many people now describe their care as "machine shop medicine." Many people complain about the cost of medicine. "It is too expensive," they say. OK, "too expensive" is a comparative so I would ask, "Too expensive compared to what?" A witch doctor? Consider the steps required to see any of the professional care providers and the number of people you deal with on any given visit:

1. Arrive at office (office space is not free, neither is the parking lot).

2. Check in (one person either sitting in front of a computer or in front of an open appointment book).

3. Vital statistics—weight, blood pressure, temperature (optional), pulse, EKG (optional) and lung function—taken by a health care professional.

4. Doctor examination (history, pathology, applicable diagnosis, medications).

5. Check out (either pay for visit or arrange for payment) and schedule next appointment (one more person sitting in front of a computer or in front of an appointment book.

In this common scenario you will have dealt with up to three health care professionals and two or more clerical support people. All are required to deliver this service for a Level One fifteen-minute visit. Who do you think has to pay for all the equipment, facilities, supplies, and people? You do. One way or another, we all do. For a patient to visit the doctor and not be prepared adds costs and burden to an already-overburdened system.

Now add to this the increasing number of patients as the population ages and the fact the doctor has only so many hours a day for being with patients. Just how many patients do you think a cardiologist can actually see a week? In a common day, a cardiologist who hustles and takes only fifteen minutes with each patient might see thirty-two people. This is a lot. But, let it take longer with a few patients and his or her whole day schedule is shot. And if there is an emergency—well, good luck in seeing the doctor any time today. As a society, we are all collectively hosed until better ways are discovered or invented. The folks who make those discoveries and create those inventions are going to be very rich.

The days of the home-visiting general practice doctor are dead. The days of the old Norman Rockwell[35] painting of the paternal doctor listening to the little girl's dolly are deader than the dolly and Norman Rockwell. Dead, dead, dead. Consider why:

- Insurance companies determine how long a doctor can spend with each patient by setting all rates
- Patient loads increase as the population ages
- Technology advancements
- New breakthroughs in treatments
- Specialization
- Skyrocketing costs
- Etc.

It is only natural to wish for a simpler time and more relaxed attitudes. In our memories, things have a tendency to seem better. Boy, it sure was better when we were younger. Right, only we didn't have any of the following:

- Preventive medicine
- Open-heart surgery
- High-technology diagnostics
- Specialization

35   **Norman Percevel Rockwell** (February 3, 1894 – November 8, 1978) was a twentieth-century American painter and illustrator. His works enjoy a broad popular appeal in the United States, where Rockwell is most famous for the cover illustrations of everyday life scenarios he created for *The Saturday Evening Post* magazine over more than four decades. Among the best-known of Rockwell's works are the *Willie Gillis* series, *Rosie the Riveter* (although his *Rosie* was reproduced less than others of the day), *Saying Grace* (1951), and the *Four Freedoms* series.

- As many sick people
- Etc., etc., etc.

If what we didn't have was the current situation, we would all be as dead as Norman Rockwell and his paternalistic doctor and the damn little girl with the cute little curl in the middle of her forehead holding the dolly. The next time you complain about how bad it is or how long you have to wait or any of the other hundred million complaints we are all capable of making, consider what the situation would be if all the new tools were never invented. I have no desire to join Norman.

In the meantime, we all have to grin and bear it. It is a damnable cost and burden. The most we have any right to expect is for the doctor to be of good heart and mean well.

Caregiver notes: Let's face it; men are complete jerks when it comes to doctors. Women, just by the fact of being women, will have had to establish an ongoing relationship with a doctor. You can't buy birth control pills over the counter, or perform in-home Pap smear tests, or get mammography down at the local drug store. Given the rapidly evolving and improving technology, someday maybe, but not today. Men, on the other hand, will go see a doctor only when something is so wrong they have no choice but to seek medical help. Given this fact, men have no idea how to establish a "doctor protocol."

Your patient may take the tried-and-true practice of having the doctor play twenty questions where the doctor tries to guess what is wrong. As the caregiver, you may not allow this. If your patient is too lazy, fearful, stubborn or spiteful to be prepared, then you must be. Wait just a darn minute. If your patient is too lazy, fearful, stubborn or spiteful to be prepared, why should you care and be prepared for him? Nuts to that. Let him know you are making the funeral preparations.

Another approach is to speak with the doctor as if your patient is not in the room and refer to him in the third person. Be prepared, your patient is not going to like this. However, when your patient finally speaks up in objection, fix him with a steely look and say, "Oh, do you wish to participate?" The only difference between a sick adult male and a sick child is…come to think of it, there is no difference between a sick adult male and a sick child.

All doctors take an oath, which may be based on the Hippocratic oath. There are many versions of this oath, the original written in ancient times and more modern ones. Graduating classes get to select which version they want to use. Here is a version written in 1964.[36]

I swear to fulfill, to the best of my ability and judgment, this covenant:

I will respect the hard-won scientific gains of those physicians in whose steps I walk, and gladly share such knowledge as is mine with those who are to follow.

I will apply, for the benefit of the sick, all measures [that] are required, avoiding those twin traps of over treatment and therapeutic nihilism.

I will remember that there is art to medicine as well as science, and that warmth, sympathy, and understanding may outweigh the surgeon's knife or the chemist's drug.

I will not be ashamed to say "I know not," nor will I fail to call in my colleagues when the skills of another are needed for a patient's recovery.

I will respect the privacy of my patients, for their problems are not disclosed to me that the world may know. Most especially must I tread with care in matters of life and death.

---

36 *Written in 1964 by Louis Lasagna, Academic Dean of the School of Medicine at Tufts University, and used in many medical schools today. Taken from the PBS Nova Web site.*

If it is given me to save a life, all thanks. But it may also be within my power to take a life; this awesome responsibility must be faced with great humbleness and awareness of my own frailty. Above all, I must not play at God.

I will remember that I do not treat a fever chart, a cancerous growth, but a sick human being, whose illness may affect the person's family and economic stability. My responsibility includes these related problems, if I am to care adequately for the sick.

I will prevent disease whenever I can, for prevention is preferable to cure.

I will remember that I remain a member of society, with special obligations to all my fellow human beings, those sound of mind and body as well as the infirm.

If I do not violate this oath, may I enjoy life and art, respected while I live and remembered with affection thereafter. May I always act so as to preserve the finest traditions of my calling and may I long experience the joy of healing those who seek my help.

Of course Hippocrates or Dr. Lasagna, are not the only ones to write a credo. Maimonides[37], a committed scholar and devoted physician who practiced in the 12th century also tried his hand. This is what he had to write:

"May I never forget that the patient is a fellow creature in pain. May I never consider him merely a vessel of disease.

---

37   **Moses Maimonides**, also known as **Rabbi Moshe ben Maimon** or the acronym the **Rambam** was born in Cordoba, Spain on March 30, 1135, and died in Egypt on December 13, 1204.[6][7]. One of the greatest Torah scholars, he was a rabbi, physician, and philosopher in Spain, Morocco and Egypt during the Middle Ages. He was the preeminent medieval Jewish philosopher. With the contemporary Muslim sage Averroes, he promoted and developed the philosophical tradition of Aristotle. As a result, Maimonides and Averroes would gain a prominent and contro-versial influence in the West, where Aristotelian thought had been lost for centuries. Albert the Great and Thomas Aquinas were notable Western readers of Maimonides.

May I have the strength, time and opportunity always to verify and correct what I have learned and to increase my understanding.

May I always be able to discover today the error of yesterday and to obtain a new light tomorrow in what I think I am sure of today."

The ancient oath swore to the god Apollo. Apollo is not a popular god these days and fell out of favor once we started to believe in a single God. However, when Hippocrates wrote the oath, he believed in supreme beings. One thing Hippocrates had in his oath was, "First to do no harm." That one line seems to have been omitted in the latter versions.

Diet

There is no doubt about it. Rating food on a scale with 1 as the lowest and 10 as the highest, I would have to award food a 42. (Will the other judges please show their cards now. Just as I thought, you all gave food a really high score.) Few pleasures in life compare with a good meal. Food is comforting and we like our comforts. I was never much of drinker (booze never was my thing) and I quit smoking when I was twenty-three. All my oral gratifications came from food. On top of this, I have never been much of a sweet eater and usually eschewed dessert, unless I was traveling and eating in fancy restaurants. Vanilla ice cream was, to me, the best dessert there was.

All of my piggish eating habits came to a screeching halt on Thursday, October 10, 2000, as did everything else in my life. I awoke at 11:00 p.m. with the worst case of indigestion I had ever had, and I have had some real beauties given my eating habits. Antacids gave me no relief so I

Yahooed heart attack symptoms and learned that, of the eight listed symptoms, I was experiencing seven. The eighth symptom was death, in which case I would not have been able to Yahoo the information.

A rhyme for my time:

I awoke that night with quite a gasp
The heartburn made me nauseous
The antacids provided no relief
Contrary to my usual belief
To the computer I went just to be cautious

The magic machine told me right then
A heart attack I was having
To the ER I fled
No wanting to be dead
Thinking my life was worth saving

The cardiologist saw me the next AM
And said these words to me:
Your valves are shot
You are not doing so hot
A surgery was meant to be

That cannot be, I said to he
I start to teach a class on Monday next
And then to Atlanta the very next week
Three thousand folks paid up to hear me speak
I have already sent the text

The cardiologist then said to me:
It is nice you're such a big shot
But your heart is completely broke
So I tell you this with no joke
You may go but come back you will not.

I went back to the Internet to get the latest greatest on heart attack symptoms. Back in the olden days of 2000, when I Yahooed for symptoms, I quickly got the eight symptoms. These days, using Google, I got a trillion or so responses with a page of "sponsored" results. I found it reassuring that someone experiencing chest pain and wanting a quick answer now has to wade through pages of sales stuff, most of which do not easily or quickly address the problem. Ain't progress great? I did eventually find a place to answer the question. Here is the answer I wanted:

Symptoms

Chest pain is a major symptom of heart attack. However, some people may have little or no chest pain, especially women, the elderly and those with diabetes. This is called a silent heart attack.

The pain may be felt in only one part of the body or move from your chest to your arms, shoulder, neck, teeth, jaw, belly area, or back.

The pain can be severe or mild. It can feel like:

- Squeezing or heavy pressure
- A tight band around the chest
- Something heavy sitting on your chest
- Bad indigestion

Pain usually lasts longer than twenty minutes. Rest and a medicine called nitroglycerine do not completely relieve the pain of a heart attack.

Other symptoms of a heart attack include:

- Shortness of breath
- Nausea or vomiting
- Anxiety

- Cough
- Fainting
- Lightheadedness—dizziness
- Palpitations (feeling like your heart is beating too fast)
- Sweating, which may be extreme

This list left out "death," which I guess is an autopsy conclusion. My cardiologist made a point of reminding me the severity of pain is not an indicator as to the severity of the heart attack. What is probably more relevant is the total number of symptoms occurring at one time. If you have a couple of the above symptoms occurring at one time, do not pass go, get yourself to the ER.

From observation, I would say most of us CAD patients are overweight. We live in this condition due to two factors: (1) we eat too much for the amount of exercise we get; and (2) we eat too many of the wrong foods, usually foods high in sugar, fat, and salt. Some potato chips would sure taste good right about now. Frito-Lay knows how good those potato chips are and sells millions and millions of tons of them a year. Those potato chips help sell soda, and it is no coincidence that PepsiCo owns Frito-Lay. Sugar, fat, and salt, mmmmm good. Can we supersize that and add a couple of burgers? Can I have an "Amen"?

A CAD clinic counselor (if your cardiologist actually has one) spends most of the time educating about the dangers of salt and fat, and for good reason. Salt causes the body to retain water and drives up blood pressure, as if your heart actually needs the extra work. Fat increases the lipid levels in your blood and those increases cause blockages of the arteries, which is why you are reading this.

Saying salt causes the body to retain water really does not explain how that unusual mechanism works. Once a person has established heart disease, subtle changes can occur in the overall contraction and/or relaxation of the heart muscle and in the resistance of the cardiovascular system's arteries. These changes put into motion a whole host of reactions in the body that results in avid retention of even more salt and water.

The body looks around and asks itself, "Where the hell can I put all this salt and water? The fluid will accumulate first in the feet and ankles. But in later stages, the fluid will also be stored in the gut wall, liver, legs and eventually the lungs. That is the problem that is seen in congestive heart failure. Think about the Great Salt Lake in Utah and the Dead Sea. The salinity in both of those bodies of water is so great a person cannot submerge. It is also almost impossible to swim in either location.

Even before one develops heart disease, too much intake of salt puts the entire cardiovascular system at risk. The salt increases the volume of the blood and now the heart must shoulder the task of pumping that increased load of fluid. The result to your system is that your blood pressure greatly escalates. Over time, the mass of the heart has to increase to meet the increased demand of the system. The larger mass of heart muscle needs more oxygen. But if the flow of blood to the heart muscle is restricted due to plaque formation in the coronary arteries...well, you know the rest. Your heart is genetically programmed to operate for some unknown amount of time. It is a machine and has a lifetime guarantee. We just don't know how long the guarantee is good for. Sears will not sell you a maintenance agreement for your heart. Like any machine, the heavier the use, the shorter the lifetime guarantees.

Apropos of nothing, the consumption of fat and salt is endemic in most cultures. Salt and fat are the two most common ingredients in those foods that taste best. The third item is sugar. Wild mammals will travel miles out of their way to get to saltlicks. In Africa, elephants have hollowed out huge caves to get to the sodium-rich dirt and travel there at least twice a year to store up all that tasty salt. In ancient Rome, soldiers received salt as part of their remuneration. This is where the word "salary" comes from.

The hunting people of Africa claimed that the best eating in the world was broiled elephant fat with salt and honey. Eating this treat caused no illness in these tribes. It is hard to have coronary disease when your primary diet is hunted lean meat and foraged fruit and vegetables and you spend so much of your life on the run. Did you ever see a fat man who depended on his hunting skills with bow and arrow and spear? That kind of fat man was usually called lion food or bait.

Diet is all about biology and, since biology is a science, it naturally follows that diet is about the laws of the science. As stated above, coronary disease is governed by Rules of Acceptance. They are Rules of Acceptance, as you can't cure the disease so you must accept it. Diet is a changing target and needs laws (not rules). And the consequence of breaking the laws is your preeminent, richly deserved, and not so unexpected death. Herewith the laws:

Science Laws

First Science Law: NO SALT! Salt is a killer. Learn to read the labels on food packages. Two thousand milligrams of salt a day for patients with CHF is the usual prescribed target. Achieving this target is not easy. The target requires vigilance and diligence. Two thousand milligrams is slightly less than one teaspoonful. This is more than adequate to keep your body functioning properly. Forget about the huge tub of popcorn at the game or the movies. As for the butter topping, your tongue should cleave to the roof of your mouth before you eat it.

Reading labels has become an art form. In the 1950s, our Congress conducted huge, well-publicized hearings into what was really going into the food we were all eating. What came out of those hearings was the pure food legislation we live with today. The straw that broke the camel's back, so to speak, was lemon cream pie. After grilling the manufacturer of the pie as to what was in the product, the truth was finally revealed. A congress-man said in his summation of the testimony: "No lemon. No cream. Just lemon cream pie." More about labels in bit.

It is not actually salt that we must avoid. It is sodium. The chemical symbol for sodium is Na. Sodium combines and chemically changes with many other chemicals and is used as a stabilizer. That means it is combined with many things to preserve freshness and enhance shelf life of everyday foods. Even foods advertised as being low salt have lots of sodium combined with substances other than chlorine.

In the 1970s, when the dangers of salt were at last being realized, a few food manufacturers decided to get into the low-salt game and began to market foods low in salt. One of the substitutes for salt these smart people came up with was sodium bromide, found in the oceans of the world in plentiful supply. One manufacturer even marketed sodium bromide in its pure form (it crystallizes just like salt) as the ultimate salt substitute. It is not as salty as salt; in fact, it is rather bitter. When the dangers of salt were finally more carefully identified as the dangers of sodium, the product was hastily pulled from the shelves.

What is interesting is that sodium and chlorine, in their pure forms, are poisons. When mixed, an atom of each to make a single salt crystal molecule, it tastes good. That molecule is 40 percent sodium and 60 percent chlorine. The biology of your body requires sodium. Sodium serves three functions:

1. Sodium is the transporter of nutrients.
2. Sodium is involved in the transmitting of nerve impulses.

3. Sodium is involved in the contractile function of muscles, including that most important muscle, the heart.

Our bodies are, after all, based on electricity, hydraulics, and chemistry. The requirement for salt makes it taste good. The body requires 250 to 500 milligrams of salt a day. That is one-sixteenth to one-eighth of a teaspoon, or as all the TV cooks say, a pinch. We just sort of overdo it. To prove the point, do this experiment:

Fill a single one-teaspoon measuring spoon with salt. This is 2,400 milligrams of salt. Now put it all in your mouth. What? You don't want to do this. I wouldn't either. Yet, if I asked you to eat three times as much but to add it a little at a time into virtually everything you eat, you would do it. I know this for a fact even though I don't know you. It is what you probably are already doing and just don't realize it.

The average American probably eats 6,000 milligrams of salt a day as an ingredient in everything. I didn't realize I was doing just this until I started to record what I was eating and listing the total salt and fat listed on labels. This meant I was eating ten to twenty times more salt a day than my body required. You are too.

To live with this law, it is necessary to learn about replacements for salt. Acquiring a taste for sour and spicy hot goes a long way in mitigating your desire for salt. Unsalted peanuts (peanuts have unsaturated fatty acids, which are long chain fatty acids that may have health benefits and are a good thing to eat in limited amounts[38]) are not only boring, they quickly lose their taste and chew appeal. Add a pinch of cayenne pepper and a dash of either ground cumin or ground oregano, and you are presented with a whole new world of chewing satisfaction. Many other varieties of nuts are extremely beneficial. The only caveat regarding

---

38   Dr. Steven Raskin, cardiologist, who also vetted the text, contributed this description of the benefit of peanuts.

nuts is to remember to eat them in limited amounts and without salt.

Pickles are wonderful if no salt is used in their preparation. Vinegar comes in many flavors and adds a flavor boost to both vegetables and meat. Vinegar may also lower blood sugar. Read the labels and make sure no salt has been added. Lemon juice and lime juice also serve as substitutes and add citrus vitamins to the mix.

In a never-ending search for a really good salt replacement it was necessary to concoct my own. I rely on flavor. Here is my recipe:

I. **Basic Rub Ingredients:** This is one of my most important basic recipes. Using only dry ingredients, this rub is for almost any meat or fish that is going to be sautéed, fried, grilled, broiled, roasted, or marinated.

    i. One heaping tablespoon of all of the following: cayenne pepper, dark chili powder, ground black pepper, both sweet and hot paprika; one-half tablespoon of garlic and onion powders, and Coleman dry mustard powder. One and one-half tablespoons of either sugar or Splenda.

    ii. To add an Italian twist to this basic recipe, do the following: omit the Coleman dry mustard powder, the dark chili powder, and cayenne pepper and replace with crushed red pepper, oregano, and basil. I leave the amounts of the new ingredients to your imagination and taste.

In many parts of the country, it is necessary to have a water softener. Water softeners work by using sodium chloride to clean the filtering elements. This adds salt to the drinking and cooking water. Not good. A replacement for salt in the filtration system is potassium chloride.

It is actually the chlorine that cleans the filter. Replacing salt with potassium chloride delivers two benefits: (1) no salt, and (2) a beneficial dose of potassium into your diet. A one-day intake of water provides the same amount of potassium as a banana. Like any of the basic minerals, it is possible to get too much potassium. We will talk more about this in the section on Renal Failure.

(I need to digress for just a moment.) Once more, I went to the Internet to do some research and found what follows. I offer it for your information:

One proven eating plan, known as the DASH diet (short for Dietary Approach to Solving Hypertension), leverages the blood pressure-reducing power of whole foods. Dash emphasizes fruits, vegetables, whole grains, and low-fat dairy foods, and limits saturated fat, cholesterol, and sodium. It is the result of a partnership between the National Institutes of Health and the American Heart Association.

When researchers from Johns Hopkins University tested the ability of diet to lower blood pressure in 459 people, they found that those who followed the dash diet for eight weeks reduced their systolic blood pressure by an average of 5.5 points and diastolic pressure by an average of 3 points. Among subjects with diagnosed hypertension, the effects were even more dramatic—dash lowered systolic pressure by 11.4 points and diastolic by 5.5 points.

One mineral that plays a key role in the dash diet is potassium. Found in substantial levels in root vegetables, leafy greens, and fruits, potassium helps balance the effects of sodium in the body. In fact, when the USDA lowered the dietary guidelines for sodium, it raised the recommendations for potassium—from 3,500 to 4,700 mg per day, a figure most of us miss. (Average potassium intakes for women hover between 2,100 to 2,300 mg, while men consume between 2,900 and 3,200 mg.) In a review of thirty-three clinical trials, researchers from Tulane University Health

Science Center in New Orleans found that increasing intake of potassium-rich foods may lower systolic blood pressure by an average of 3 points and diastolic by 2 points.

One out of every four Americans has high blood pressure, also known as hypertension. (By age sixty-five, half of all adult Americans have hypertension). Although lifestyle changes can help—such as being physically active and quitting smoking—when it comes to diet, most people think lowering sodium intake is the most important change they can make. But studies suggest a team of minerals—including sodium, calcium, magnesium, and potassium—keeps the heart pumping smoothly and blood pressure on an even keel.

Potassium, however, could be the key. Researchers found that a diet full of potassium-rich foods, such as orange juice, raisins, and sweet potatoes, may actually blunt the effects of too much sodium. In the landmark study on diet and blood pressure called DASH (Dietary Approaches to Stop Hypertension), volunteers who ate nine to eleven servings of fruits and vegetables per day, three servings of low-fat dairy foods, and lower amounts of sodium were able to decrease their blood pressure within two weeks. Researchers speculate that one of the primary reasons for these dwindling numbers was a high intake of potassium.

In addition to keeping blood pressure in check, potassium helps regulate the balance of fluid in the body to help prevent muscle cramps. That's why athletes who work out in hot, humid climates often reach for potassium-rich food, such as a banana or orange juice, after a hard workout.

The latest guidelines released by the Institute of Medicine encourage Americans to aim for 4.7 grams (or 4,700 milligrams) of this blood pressure–lowering mineral each day. And food is the best way to get the potassium you need. (In rare cases, a doctor may prescribe a potassium supplement for patients taking diuretics.) Most fruits and vegetables, and even beef and fish, are high in potassium.

(This was copied as it was printed and I am not responsible for the errors in spelling, capitalization, or punctuation; I have enough trouble getting my own stuff right. It seems the more we learn the more we need to learn. Don't you just hate that when it happens? Worse for me, I forgot to notate where I found this wonderful short piece. You will have to forgive me for not attributing this.)

After I had added all the above about the importance of potassium, one of the doctors vetting the book pointed out that patients suffering from kidney disease have to be very careful of their potassium intake. Those renal patients need to be aware of the risks of potassium. I went to look it up to find out why. My thought was to add that information. No such luck. However, what did occur was the requirement to write about renal failure as it relates to heart disease. In that section, which appears later in this book, I explain exactly how it all works.

Once you acquire the taste for hot, you will find nothing can replace it. Hot makes foods fairly sparkle with flavor. Bless the hot pepper and the sauces made from them. Hot salsa, mmmmmmm. Great on everything. Where we get in trouble with salsa is when we eat it with chips. Salty, fat-fried chips and salsa are a natural go together. Americans eat more salsa a year than they eat ketchup. This is quite an accomplishment given the huge number of hamburgers and servings of French fries we eat.

Alan Alda[39] of *MASH* fame used to have a science program on PBS. Alda had one show where the subject of taste was the topic. He was attending one of the many great food

---

39   **Alan Alda** (born **Alphonso Joseph D'Abruzzo**; January 28, 1936) is an American actor, director and screenwriter. He is best known for his role as Hawkeye Pierce in the TV series *M*A*S*H*. During the 1970s and 1980s, he was viewed as the archetypal sympathetic male, though in recent years, he has appeared in roles that counter that image.

contests held in Texas and was sampling the super hot salsas. Before sampling the habanero salsas, he said he could handle very hot foods because he had a "bitter" mouth. With CAD, this is something to be devoutly wished for.

Second Science Law: NO FAT! If the salt doesn't get you, the fat will. Cholesterol is an insidious killer. Cholesterol will silently build up in your arteries and molecule-by-molecule block off and shut down the mechanism of getting the blood circulating. The weakened and sick veins will never complain or give you any warning. However, sooner than later, the heart is going to notice it does not get enough oxygen and it will kill itself by causing muscle tissue to die. Now, this hurts. And not just a little bit. As you probably know, heart attacks hurt, a lot.

Also, contrary to popular belief, cholesterol does not just collect and form inside the blood vessels. It also collects in the walls of the arteries. The medical term for this is atherosclerosis. This is "the" term you do not want to hear applied to you. If not discovered, it will quietly build and build in the wall, and when enough cholesterol collects, it will either shut down the line or cause the line to erupt. This is not a desirable condition.

Specifically, this is what happens. Over time your body stores low-density lipids in the walls of the lines (arteries and veins) delivering blood to the heart muscle. Noticing the irritation in the wall, the body sends white blood cells to the area to kill the demon irritation. The only problem is there is no place for the lipids to disperse to so the combination of the lipids and the white blood cells form a bigger mass called plaque. Eventually the wall can no longer hold the entire mass and it ruptures. The severity of the rupture determines how much longer you have to live.

The other impact of the growing mass of plaque both inside the wall and inside the artery is the gradual closing of the vessel without causing a rupture in the wall. This will eventually close the artery down and stop blood flow to the heart. The medical term for this condition is stenosis. This condition leads to all the bypass surgeries. And that is painful. You got a pain in your chest, get to the ER.

Dr. Peter Libby, Chief of Cardiovascular Medicine and Mallinckrodt Professor of Medicine, Brigham and Women's Hospital and the Harvard Medical School, in an article that appeared in the New York Times on April 8, 2007, said the process is comprised of the following six steps:

- LDL cholesterol (the bad fat) particles are absorbed by the artery wall, prompting cells in the wall to summon the immune system.
- White blood cells of the immune system travel to the irritation and squeeze into the artery wall.
- The white blood cells send out chemical signals that cause inflammation.
- The white blood cells grow and start to ingest the LDL particles. This is the start of pimple like growths called plaque.
- As the plaque enlarges it is covered with a cap of smooth muscle cells.
- Eventually this cap ruptures into the bloodline and attracts red blood cells. The red cells form a clot to seal the surface of the plague. However, the clot can grow and may eventually block the artery. This block causes the heart attack.

∽

Learning the substitution game is a bit tricky. About six years ago, during the great fat and carbohydrate scares (which would cause the value of Krispy Kreme[40] stock to fall through the floor), the food manufacturers figured out how to get into the new game. The manufacturers started to produce and market foods "low in fat." Entenmann's Bakery,[41] being no dummies, quickly came to market with a new line of fat pills, er, doughnuts, advertised to contain 30 percent less fat.

This was good news to doughnut lovers everywhere, among whom I count myself (funny, I never was a police officer). What they did was simple. They made the doughnuts a third smaller. They did not change a single ingredient. Not one. It was only by carefully reading the portion size that my wife showed me what the secret was. This is a common ploy. Food makers simply change the portion size to accommodate the fad or worry of the day.

Here is as good a place as any to talk about portion size as it pertains to food levels of salt and fat. Food manufacturers keep changing portion sizes to comply with best eating habits, or at least, appear to comply. Once you get the hang of reading the labels, you will notice that portion sizes as recommended on the labels have no basis in reality. I don't think I have ever eaten a quarter cup of anything. A quarter cup is two ounces. TWO OUNCES! I never saw anyone eat only two ounces of nuts or cheese or peanut butter. And worse, over the years, as our expanding waistlines demonstrated, a portion size was entirely contingent on our appetites.

40   **Krispy Kreme** is a chain of doughnut stores. Its parent company is **Krispy Kreme Doughnuts, Inc.** (NYSE: KKD), based in Winston-Salem, North Carolina, United States. Krispy Kreme sells a variety of doughnuts, among them its traditional glazed doughnut, often served warm. As Krispy Kreme fans the world over will attest nothing is better than a warm, fresh glazed Krispy Kreme. This last sentence is an editorial comment.

41   **Entenmann's**, is a company that manufactures and delivers sweet baked goods. The company offers dessert cakes, donuts, ultimates, cookies, loaf breads, pies, club packs, singles, cereal bars, little bites, Enten-mini's products, as well as Danish, crumb cakes, and buns.

Fast-food franchises continually upped portion sizes and introduced "supersizing." We weight over-advantaged folks have come to believe that a portion size is a supersize. That is what we order and that is what we eat, whether we need to or not. It is very important that you get the hang of the difference between your portion size and the label portion size.

When I was a kid—you might remember those halcyon days of yore—a cigar cost a nickel and if you got caught smoking one your father tanned your backside, a Coke (the real thing) came in an eight-ounce green bottle. Find one of those today, I dare you. Nope, today Coke comes in a pint or twenty-ounce bottle. The calories were not listed on that eight-ounce green bottle. If the calories had been listed, there might have been around 120. Today's twenty-ounce bottle has in excess of 250 calories. Check it out.

A good question might be "Just how much fat a day can I eat?" Cardiologists recommend your diet should contain not more than 30 percent fat. In a 2000 calorie-a-day diet this equates to 600 fat calories. The other issue regarding fat is whether the fat is LDL (bad) or HDL (good) fat. And how does this relate to portion size?

If we look back over the past twenty years, we can get a better appreciation of how supersizing has helped increase out waist sizes and cholesterol levels. A generation ago, the hamburger served was 300 plus calories and made from meat that was 80 percent lean (more about that in a moment). Today, the burger is larger, made from 70 or 75 percent lean, and weighs in at a hefty 600 calories.

The natural go-with for the burger is, of course, French fries. The serving side of fries has grown from two and half ounces to almost seven ounces. Calories have tripled from approximately two hundred to six hundred. The amount of salt has had to increase to keep pace with this expansion, as did the amount of ketchup. More spuds fried in fat, more salt and ketchup with more salt and more sugar. Life is so good.

In that same time span, the portion size of that all-American favorite, spaghetti, grew from one cup of pasta with sauce and three small meatballs providing five hundred or so calories to today's stevedore-size portion of two cups of pasta with meat sauce, three large meatballs, over one thousand calories and a doggy bag. The plates the restaurants use have grown in size to accommodate this growth. Big plates piled high with food—it's the American way. (I wonder if this is what Superman[42] had in mind when he fought for Truth, Justice, and the American Way.)

Here is a short list of common foodstuffs and their before and after sizes:[43]

Item	Size and Calories Before	Size and Calories After
Coffee (Sweet /Milk)	8 oz, 45 cal	Mocha 16 oz, 350 cal
Muffin	1.5 oz, 210 cal	4 oz, 500 cal
Pepperoni Pizza Slice	500 cal	850 cal
Popcorn	5 cups, 270 cal	11 cups, 630 cal
Bagel	3-inch diameter, 140 cal	6-inch diameter, 350 cal

What the raw numbers do not include are the increased amounts of sodium and fat we have added to our diets. For instance, the bagel, as eaten in many parts of the country, is

---

42 **Superman** is a fictional character, a comic book superhero widely considered to be an American cultural icon. Created by American writer Jerry Siegel and Canadian-born artist Joe Shuster in 1932 while both were living in Cleveland, Ohio, and sold to Detective Comics, Inc., in 1938, the character first appeared in *Action Comics* #1 (June 30, 1938) and subsequently appeared in various radio serials, television programs, films, newspaper strips, and video games.

43 Statistics from the American Heart Association and Banner Boswell Hospital, Sun City, Arizona.

not a bagel until it has the "schmear." The schmear is a thick layer of cream cheese, sometimes with lox, sometimes without. The schmear with lox adds on both the salt and the fat.

The real money made by theaters is not just the price of admission but the concession stands. What is a movie without the popcorn and soda? The movie folks even offer you a deal. Buy the big, big, big tub of popcorn and the big, big, big soda and you can get a free refill of both. Want butter with that? Of course, and make that double, double, double butter, please. The butter is not really butter, as that would be too expensive. It is usually a trans fat (LDL bad fat) substitute. And while we are at, an extra sprinkle or two or three of the flavored salt would be nice. We like to do things in a big, big, big way.

Third Science Law: LEARN ABOUT SUBSTITUTION. Ice cream and butter must go the way of the dodo bird. For me, taking red meat out of my diet was the real killer. But I did it. It was not easy. When I get a craving for red meat that I can't assuage, I go eat a buffalo burger. Smothered in hot sauce under a heap of raw onion is as close to red meat nirvana as I am going to get. (And hold the salt, please.)

Sitting at home, watching television, is the great American exercise routine. The exercise comes from the almost nonstop snacking that accompanies the watching and is called elbow bends. What is better than potato chips and dips? The snack food industry (hello, PepsiCo again) knows salt and fat are the most essential ingredients to the snack foods and provide what seems to be an infinite number of varieties. There are literally varieties for every taste and preference. How many different flavors of sour cream are there? Lots!

If you don't like fish now, you had better learn to love it. Salmon, herring, and mackerel are super rich in omega-3 oils. You can make each day a little bit brighter by eating a little pickled herring by Vita. White meat chicken, turkey breast, and pork (the other white meat) are the other items that round out my diet. Suffice it to say, the pork must be surgically cleaned of all visible fat. Lately, fresh buffalo, sometimes labeled as bison, has been added as an infrequent item in a local store. Glory, glory halleluiah, this means guilt-free red meat. Buffalo has twenty-five percent of the fat of beef. Buffalo cooks in about forty percent of the time beef does.

It is impossible to remove all fats from your diet, nor should you, and anyone proposing such a thing must be smoking some seriously strange substances. However, it is not unreasonable to limit your intake to less than 30 percent caloric value of your daily diet. Once again, due vigilance and diligence are required. You can do it. Your life depends on it.

Now for some really good news: For every one milligram of extra HDL calories you eat a day, you receive an automatic decrease of two milligrams of LDL. If you start to get your cholesterol total readings under 200 and increase your HDL levels to 40 and above, watch what happens to your total cholesterol. It will astound you.

I have discovered a silver bullet to help drastically reduce my LDL count. It is not oatmeal. It is factual that oatmeal can help lower LDL. However, the commercials do not say reduces LDL. It says it reduces your total cholesterol count. Also factual, but in and of itself it doesn't quite explain exactly how this miracle is achieved. Think about it for a minute. What is the great American breakfast? Smoked and fried pig meat and eggs with hot buttered toast and fried potatoes and, in some restaurants, some pancakes! All of this food is yours for under $8 (where is my fork and knife?). Part of the miracle is the substitution for all that cholesterol found in those foods with a grain. Well, duh. The oatmeal diet will also help you lose weight. Again, well, duh.

Oatmeal has 1 percent soluble fiber. The soluble fiber carries off the fat. You can eat many other things that have two or three times the soluble fiber. Beans are rich in not only soluble fiber but also protein. Beans can be used as a replacement for meat and many cultures that are in short supply of meat eat diets rich in beans of all types, colors, and flavors. By a strange circumstance, those cultures have thin people that are well nourished. You will also find that by replacing meat with high-protein beans you will lower your overall grocery bill. Lowering our grocery bills is not a very high priority with most Americans. Salty, fatty snacks are expensive and look how much of that stuff we eat.

Green vegetables are good providers of soluble fiber, especially the greens from the cabbage family. Broccoli, green cabbage, and Chinese cabbages (Napa and bok choy), to name just a few, are all rich in soluble fiber. Many fruits are also great providers. Oranges, apples (all pomes), bananas, and mangos top the list for me. These fruits also provide healthy doses of potassium, another of the essential minerals your body requires.

Take seriously the recommendation to eat five fresh fruits and vegetables a day. Fried potatoes are not on the list. As a side note to vegetables—dark bitter greens are very high in iron. In fact, the more bitter the green, the more iron it probably contains. When you eat lots of greens, you must tell your INR[44] nurse. Vegetables high in iron will distort your INR levels.

The silver bullet is a fish oil capsule. I take two a day. This is a big dose. But I sometimes take more. Whenever I eat anything that I think might exceed my maximum daily requirement for fat, I take another cap, usually with that meal. The fish oil acts like red wine and forces the body to expel the extra fat. Now, as a matter of fact, I don't know if a cardiologist would recommend this approach. However,

---

44   The prothrombin time (PT or protime) test is used to calculate your international normalized ratio (INR). Your INR will help your health care provider determine how fast your blood is clotting and whether your medication dose needs to be changed. Illness, diet, medication changes, and physical activities may affect your INR. WebMD

my cholesterol level is 147 with my HDL count over sixty. The approach works for me. **Now the limit of liability statement: You should not automatically adopt this approach without careful consultation with your doc and your counselor.**

I went to the American Heart Association to get some idea about how much fat is really in the food we eat. The American Heart Association has scads of information on the subject of diet and I was able to glean (read that "steal") the following table:

Fat Examples

Item	Size	Fat Grams	Amount/Tsp
Hamburger 80%	3 oz	15	3
Hamburger 95%	3 oz	6	1
Beef Hot Dog	1 ea	13	3
Lite Hot Dog	1 ea	2.5	0.5
Whole Milk 4%	8 oz	6	2
French Fries	Medium	25	5
Chicken Nuggets	6 pcs	20	4
Deep Dish Pizza extra cheese	Medium Slice	17	3.5
Thin Crust Pizza	Medium Slice	8	2
Ham, Egg, Cheese Biscuit	1	24	5
Whole Wheat Toast	1	2.5	0.5
Vanilla Ice Cream	.5 cup	7	1.5
Cheddar Cheese	1 oz	9	2
Mozzarella Cheese	1 oz	4.5	1
Potato Chips	1 oz	11	2.5
Turkey Ham	1 oz	1.5	0.5
Ranch Dressing	2 tbsp	16	3.5
Hummus	2 tbsp	2.5	0.5
Baked Potato	1	0.25	0
Fat-Free Milk	8 oz	0	0
Frozen Fat-Free Yogurt	.5 cup	0	0
Pop Corn, Air Popped	1 cup	0.5	0

This is not meant to be an all-inclusive table of everything you may eat. It is offered only as an example. If you don't agree with the numbers, please get in touch with the American Heart Association. I am only the reporter.

Fourth Science Law: GET EDUCATED. Learn what is good for you, and avoid what is not. This can be rather depressing. Most of the foods you really like are going to be on a "do not eat" list. Almost all ethnic foods are going to be on the list. Chinese food, at least the way it is prepared in this country, is about as bad for you as you can get. It relies on large doses of MSG (mono**sodium** glutamate) to enhance or bring out the flavors of the food. Chinese food relies on soy sauce to supply the salty flavor. About the only thing higher in sodium is salt itself.

Finding a good substitute for salt was very difficult. I have found one. I rely on flavor. Here is the recipe for a rub I concocted to replace salt:

- **Basic Rub Ingredients**. This is one of my most important basic recipes. Using only dry ingredients, this rub is for almost any meat or fish that is going to be sautéed, fried, grilled, broiled, roasted, or marinated.
  - One heaping tablespoon of all of the following: cayenne pepper, dark chili powder, ground black pepper, both sweet and hot paprika; one-half tablespoon of garlic and onion powders and Coleman dry mustard powder. One and one-half tablespoons of either sugar or Splenda.
  - To add an Italian twist to this basic recipe, do the following: Omit the Coleman dry mustard powder, the dark chili powder, and cayenne pepper and replace with crushed red pepper, oregano and basil. I leave the

amounts of the new ingredients to your imagination and taste.

You may have noticed this is the second time I give you this recipe. It is with intent I do so. Getting salt out of your diet is so important I thought it appropriate to repeat the recipe.

Fifth Science Law: EASTABLISH AND STICK TO YOUR DIET. Many CAD patients take blood thinners to prevent blood clots. This is especially true if you have a stent or mechanical valves in your heart. Clots can gum up mechanical valves but that's not the real problem. What you worry about is the clots building up on the valve then breaking off and traveling to the brain (stroke) or lungs (pulmonary embolism), either of which can be permanently debilitating or deadly.[45] If a clot blocks and gums up a valve, you probably have about seven minutes to live. Don't worry about this even though a blocked valve is going to be very painful. You will probably pass out in three minutes or so and you won't know you are dying. I know this is cold comfort but I am making a point here. Watch your INR.

Clots don't gum up a valve but they can build up there and then get thrown to the brain (stroke) or lungs (pulmonary embolism) either of which can be permanently debilitating or deadly.[46]

Blood thinners are affected by changes in diet. If you don't usually drink and you decide to have a couple of beers at the game, your INR is going to be affected. Have a hankering for green vegetables that is above your normal intake, INR will be skewed. When the technician asks you if there are any changes at the start of your INR test, tell

---

45 Dr. Mark Moeller, Family Practice.

46 Dr. Mark Moeller, M.D. Family Practice, Sutter West Medical Group, Davis, Ca.

the technician about diet changes. This is need-to-know information.

I am not going to write any more about fats and cholesterol. Your cardiac counselor is far more qualified than I to explain how high- and low-density lipids work. What I can do that the counselor can't is give you practical advice on how to cope as a surviving open-heart surgery patient. What gives me the right to write about these issues is I have had two open-heart surgeries to replace both my aortic and mitral valves and a four-way bypass. I have no natural heartbeat and I am 100 percent dependent on a pacemaker. The point is that almost anything you have done that could be bad for you, I have done. Following the rules allows me to be here to tell you what I have learned. And now practice.

I learned something new when Tim Russert[47] died. Tim appeared, on camera, to be in good health. Not so. He suffered from heart disease and diabetes (the deadly duo), was a workaholic, and a driven man. He had only one heart attack. It was all that he needed to have. A new statistic was released, at least new to me. It has to do with waist size.

It appears that all that lard we carry around in the middle of our bodies is really deadly. Women with waist sizes greater than thirty-five inches and men with waist sizes greater than forty inches increase their chances of heart disease exponentially to those with smaller waist girths. The waist size for Asians is set even lower. This is the surrogate for what is called visceral fat. It is the fat between abdominal organs; this is the dangerous fat. The subcutaneous fat—that's the loose flab just under the skin that a plastic surgeon charges big bucks for to do liposuction.

---

47 Timothy John Russert (May 7, 1950 – June 13, 2008) was an American television journalist and lawyer who appeared for more than sixteen years as the longest-serving moderator of NBC's *Meet the Press*.

There has been much discussion in this book and there is soooo much on the Web about diet. I went and did some research, not much, to learn just how much stuff there is. I did a search on Amazon to find out how many books there are about cooking. I did both a generic search just to see how many cookbooks there are and a specific search for diet books specifically for heart disease.

Amazon lists mere˙ 1,033 titles for heart disease diets, many from the American Heart Association (well, I guess they should know). When it comes to cookbooks in general Amazon lists 103,000 titles. I further queried books that were about eating. I was rewarded by being informed Amazon has over 600,000 titles they will be happy to sell you so you can learn how to eat. This does not include all the books that might be in and out of print.

When I asked Amazon how many books they sold on dieting they reported back they had a few—21,000. Now, if you are looking for a dieting program cookbook, how is a person supposed to find the right one? I want a diet that will help me maintain and won't make me feel like I never will enjoy a meal again. How about if I want to eat out? As they say in Brooklyn, "Fuggedaboutit."

My inescapable conclusion to these numbers: Folks like to eat and cook. Folks do not like to diet.

Medications

Americans in general and sick Americans in particular, have become indoctrinated to the philosophy that a pill can cure anything and everything. I tried to count the number of commercials on TV that claimed that this or that advertised pill would absolutely make you feel better. What is most interesting is that the commercials are for medications that require a prescription. Strange, huh?

I wonder how many doctors are besieged by patients demanding they dispense prescriptions for the latest wonder pills.

Taking the daily meds becomes, not unlike a religious doctrine, a daily ritual. To facilitate the many times daily of drug taking, many patients start their day by counting out all the drugs needed for the day and putting them in a compartmentalized container. These drug containers come in a variety of sizes and accommodate the smallest to the largest pills and capsules. Some religions face east several times a day and pray. We face the container several times a day and take those drugs. Amen. Like religious cant, we don't ask why we are taking the pills any more than religious supplicants question why a prayer is said. We are sick, we live in the cathedral of medicine, and the drugs are our ritual.

We are obsessed with medicine. We are as obsessed with medicine as we are with food. We wallow in our illnesses and take another pill or two. We look for new sicknesses we can have and, when a new drug is announced, we pounce on it and run off to the doctor to get a prescription. For example, I didn't even know there was a disease like restless leg syndrome until there was a pill to cure it. What ever happened to Doan's Little Liver Pills?

I was wondering just how rampant our dependence on prescription medications has become. I know in my case I kind of liked the idea I had to take so many medications and I will talk about that later. Then lo and behold, an article appeared that answered that exact question. Well, I just could just not stop myself from sharing the information with you. I print it exactly as it appeared. I will even include that part of the article that addresses the issues of emotional dependency although that issue is addressed in some significant detail in the section on depression, anxiety and depression.

America's Most Medicated States
Prescription drug rates are highest in places where preventable chronic diseases are the norm.
By Rebecca Ruiz, Forbes on MSN.com

"Much of the American South is ailing, with West Virginia the worst off—at least, if the rate of prescription drug use is any indication. The state filled 17.7 prescriptions per capita compared to a national average of 11.5, according to Verispan, a health care information company.

Alabama, South Carolina, Tennessee, Arkansas, Louisiana, Kentucky and Missouri also have prescription drug-use rates well above the national average.

"The growth in prescription drug use," says Barlow, is driven in part by "chronic diseases that are largely preventable and are linked to lifestyle and physical activity."

Behind the Trends

In 2008, total sales for prescription drugs reached $291.5 billion, a 1.4 percent increase from the previous year. Lipitor, a statin used to control cholesterol, was the top-selling drug, followed by the acid reflux medication Nexium, and Plavix, an anti-platelet agent that reduces the risk of heart attack or stroke. Sales of cardiovascular and gastroenterology medications, as well as ones that regulate central nervous system issues like seizures, depression, pain and Alzheimer's, accounted for half of all drug sales in 2008.

Verispan's data are gathered from retail pharmacies but exclude those filled by mail order, which comprised 7 percent of prescriptions filled in 2007.

The most prescribed drug to Medicare beneficiaries in West Virginia in 2007, according to the Centers for Medicare and Medicaid Services, was lisinopril, a generic drug used to treat high blood pressure. West Virginians have higher rates of heart-disease death: 237 per 100,000 compared to a national average of 200.

And their health problems don't end there. Twelve percent of the population has diabetes, nearly 4 percent more than the average rate. Worse yet, almost 70 percent of West Virginians are obese or overweight, more than one-quarter smoke and 30 percent report having poor mental health, according to the Centers for Disease Control and Prevention.

John Law, a spokesman for the state's department of health and human services, says public health officials are attempting to improve these statistics through a number of measures, including smoking-prevention programs for teenagers, more funding of mental health facilities and promoting healthy lifestyle choices such as eating nutritious food and getting exercise.

Mental Wellness

Though physical inactivity is clearly linked to prescription drug trends, poor mental health has also influenced usage patterns: Antidepressants were the third most-popular type of drug dispensed in 2008, with $9.5 billion in sales.

The percentage of non-elderly adults who used antidepressants increased from 6 percent to 10 percent between 1996 and 2005, according to Dr. Mark Olfson, a professor of clinical psychiatry at Columbia University Medical Center who recently analyzed these trends and published the findings in the *Journal of the American Medical Association*.

Olfson and his co-author, Steven C. Marcus, a professor at the University Pennsylvania School of Social Policy & Practice, found that the increase occurred regardless of gender, age, marital status, educational level and health insurance status.

Despite the increase in antidepressant use, Olfson says it's unclear if the trend indicates that more Americans are struggling with mental health issues. Rather, Olfson cites the growing acceptance of discussing and treating depression and the use of antidepressants for conditions like insomnia and back pain as factors for the increase.

Heightened awareness of certain drugs and conditions may be another explanation. In 2005, pharmaceutical companies spent $122 million on direct-to-consumer anti-depressant advertising—almost four times what they spent in 1999. A 2005 study in *JAMA*, The Journal of the American Medical Association, found that 55 percent of participants who requested a brand-name drug received an antide-pressant; only 10 percent of patients who had similar symp-toms but made no request received an antidepressant.

Finally, fewer patients are seeing psychotherapists to resolve their mental health problems. Instead, says Olfson, "there's a greater emphasis on drugs."

That seems to be true regardless of which preventable condition is being treated.

John Law acknowledges that West Virginia's prescrip-tion rate is high, but says the combination of lifestyle changes and appropriate medication can only help improve a patient's condition.

"We're working diligently to turn that around," Law says, referring to the prevalence of chronic disease in the state. "But you don't turn that around in a year—it takes a long time.""

I particularly liked that last "Not my fault" statement. Of course you can't turn it around in a year. In order to fix such a horrific situation it is necessary to start to educate the population at an early age.

If you find yourself reading just how much money the pharmaceutical companies spend on advertising to induce you to buy their drugs, and you start to get angry, well, welcome to the club. What are you going to do about it? The first thing you can do is to start questioning the value of the meds you are taking and why you are taking them. We will write more on this in the depression section.

Thinking about how quick we are to take a pill required some interesting rules. I call these Prescription Proscriptions.

Prescription Proscriptions

Proscription One: Know what you are taking and why. Education, education, education.

Proscription Two: Take the medications as prescribed. I have met patients that have halved the amount of some of the drugs they take. The reason they give is "cost." Drugs are damn expensive and Medicare Part D does not cover all the costs. This makes med costs onerous. In the section on testing, we discussed how dosages are arrived at. When you arbitrarily decrease the amount of any given drug, it has a "ripple" effect. Other drugs you take may be dependent on the drug you reduced. The effect of this is you are now taking two ineffective drugs instead of one. Halving or reducing amount negates the positive effect of the drug. There is a reason why medications are prescribed the way they are. You can't run the risk of ignoring the directions. Wait a minute, I take that back. You can always run the risk of ignoring the directions; that is why it is called "risk."

Proscription Three: All drugs are toxic and may have side effects. Watch for side effects when taking any drug. Drugs also have interactions with other drugs. For this reason alone it is wise to get all your medications from a single source. Pharmacists in the United States are mandated to check for any possible conflicts between drugs.

Proscription Four: Drugs are not "bulletproof" vests. Just because you take a drug does not mean you can forget about other courses of treatment. For instance, taking a drug to reduce cholesterol does not mean you can eat fat. If you are not going to follow all the treatment rules, don't follow any.

Proscription Five: If something changes, immediately tell your doctor. Taking a drug for a while does not mean you will not suddenly develop a serious side effect. Some side effects may be gradual and may not be "sudden," so if you do feel different, tell your doc. **If you feel different, tell your doc.**[48]

Proscription Six: Make sure you renew your prescriptions in plenty of time so they do not run out. The last thing you need is to find yourself in a crisis mode because you did not renew in time. Ask if your pharmacy has automatic "reminders," or use one of the devices out there that function as reminders. Some folks need aids and if you need memory aids use them so you will not run out of medications.

Proscription Seven: Do not start arbitrarily taking any over-the-counter medications. There is no such thing as an innocuous drug. If you have a cold or some other ailment and are looking for symptomatic relief, call your primary care provider. In some cases, your pharmacist can give you the best guidance. The pharmacist knows what drugs you are taking (most especially true if you get all your meds from one place), and can help select the best option for

---

48 Krishna Schiller, PharmD, clinical pharmacist, Banner Good Samaritan Hospital, Phoenix, Arizona.

you. It was pointed out to me that a good pharmacist is helpful for selecting appropriate cold remedies. If you choose to follow the advice of a pharmacist, inform your primary care provider and your cardiologist.[49] Your care provider will know what you are taking and will either prescribe or recommend something that will not cause you any interaction problem.

Proscription Eight: Carry a current and updated list of all your drugs, dosages, and directions at all times when you are out and about. In an emergency, this list could save your life. This is especially important if you take blood thinners and high blood pressure medications.

Proscription Nine: Herbal remedies, supplements, and teas are drugs. We don't think of these items as drugs but they are. In sufficient quantity, they can be toxic. What is even subtler is their potential interaction with prescription medications. The most common side effects are the interactions with blood thinners, hypertension drugs, and mood-modifying medications.[50]

There is now even a new diagnosis for male heart attack victims. It is an ED coronary. The men who are the victims of this coronary have heard the advertisement for Viagra or another such drug and have found a way to get some. Every one of the advertisements warns against a priapism, an erection lasting for more than four hours. That condition sounds like a good deal to them so they find a method to get a few of the blue pills, sometimes on the black market. These guys I put in the same class as smokers—complete morons.

---

49 Ibid.
50 Ibid.

One medication that is usually prescribed for a heart patient is a sleeping drug. Once again, contrary to the advertisements, sleep drugs are, in fact, addictive. There is a worse dependency than physical dependency. It is a psychological dependency. This goes back to our indoctrination about pills.

Far worse for the patient is reliance on a pill to improve or to relieve the depression. I will discuss this in the section on depression.

One of the more commonly prescribed medications for those suffering with chronic heart failure is a diuretic. Diuretics are not prescribed for all CAD sufferers. "Water pills," as some call them, should be called urine pills. A byproduct of CHF is the buildup of fluid in the lung tissue because of failure of the left ventricle to effectively pump blood. As the condition worsens, there is a greater stimulus for the body to retain even more fluid. In severe circumstances, it is possible for the body to add several pounds of water weight a day. If things get bad enough, you could conceivably drown in your own juices.

As the amount of water increases in the lungs, breathing becomes more and more labored. A chest X-ray will show the severity of the excess fluid. Sometimes the fluid becomes sequestered within the body cavity around the lungs, a condition called a pleural effusion. One of the procedures used to drain off this excess fluid is a thoracentesis.

A pulmonary doctor usually performs this procedure. You must remain awake and upright for this procedure. The doctor will insert a needle through your rib cage in your back and penetrate the lining. The needle is attached by way of a tube to a vacuum bottle. When the lining is pierced, the vacuum will automatically suck out all the fluid. Relief is immediate. In the grand scheme of things, a thoracentesis is not very painful. It is a tad uncomfortable.

One of the pulmonary specialists[51] that vetted this work thought a slightly longer explanation was required. I am quoting, directly: "After a CABG,[52] patients can get pleural effusions called 'post pericardiectomy effusions.' These are not uncommon after surgical procedures involving the pericardium. These are thought to be inflammatory in etiology.[53] They are drained, if larger, and treatment for reoccurrence is prednisone or other drug."

When the liquid amount becomes immense enough, the body will look for new places to store the fluids. The body, having the miraculous nature of its engineering

being compromised, will take the path of least resistance and put that fluid in your feet and lower legs. The body is going to find some place to store the fluid. The more obese you are, the more places there are to store the fluid.

Either your cardiologist or internist will monitor your care while taking these drugs. One of the many tests they perform concerns your feet and ankles. Every visit, regardless of how long a time you are under their care, they will look

---

51 Dr. Shannon Valenzuela, Pulmonary Disease

52 **Coronary artery bypass surgery,** also **coronary artery bypass graft surgery,** and colloquially **heart bypass** or **bypass surgery,** is a surgical procedure performed to relieve angina and reduce the risk of death from coronary artery disease

53 **–noun, plural -gies.**
1. *Pathology.*
    a. The study of the causes of diseases.
    b. The cause or origin of a disease.

2. The study of causation.
3. Any study of causes, causation, or causality, as in philosophy, biology, or physics.
    Based on the Random House Unabridged Dictionary, © Random House, Inc. 2006

at and feel your ankles. They are judging how puffy you are. The scale used goes from 0 to +4.0 is normal. The progression is geometric. Plus one is a mild puffiness. Plus 2 is twice as much puffiness as plus one. Plus 3 is twice plus 2, and plus 4 is twice plus 3. Got it?

There is a degree of expansion even worse than plus 4. In this case, the water retention is so great the lower leg cannot contain it. The skin bursts from the pressure and the legs ooze or seep the fluid. This is very akin to a hot dog splitting from the water expansion on the grill. This makes a yummy hot dog but a terrible medical condition.

If you don't understand the engineering, it does not matter. It only matters to say you are now really, really sick. If you have this problem, it means you are not taking very good care of yourself. Like a smoker, you are not following the protocols. Please stop coming to see your doctor. Go off somewhere and die on your own dollar.

From years of experience, I can tell you exactly what life is like on diuretics. The worse your CHF, the worse the problem you will have with water retention and the more reliant you will be on the use of the diuretics. I made a list of the things you need to know:

1. Take your diuretic in the morning. Lasix (probably the most commonly prescribed drug) lasts six hours, just like its name.

2. The drug can take anywhere from thirty minutes to one hour to start to work.

3. Once the drug takes effect, you will have to urinate every thirty to forty minutes. Sometimes the interval is a little longer.

4. This is a pain in the ass.

5. You must weigh yourself every day and you must keep a record of your morning weight. Weigh yourself after you have voided in the morning and record this weight.

6. If you gain more than four pounds over a one-week period, call your doctor.

7. Do not try to travel while you are taking this drug. Forget about flying. You must stay in your seat for long periods and you don't want to risk an accident.

8. If running errands, plan your shopping around thirty-minute intervals between restrooms.

9. This is a pain in the ass.

10. When you dine out, sit at the end of the table. You will have to get up often during the meal and you want to minimize disturbing your company.

11. Don't go the movies while the drug is working. You will probably have to go during the most important scene. Also, the other theatergoers will kick your ass for disturbing them.

12. You will know when the drug is wearing off. I can't really describe it, but you will notice a change in the color.and nature of your urine. You will probably think that you will expel more fluid the last time the pill works. Another indication might be a sense of tightness in your calves and ankles as if your muscles have been wrung dry. This is different for everyone.

13. Take note of how your body is reacting to these drugs. Over a short period, you will start to know what is appropriate and what is not. When things seem to get out of bounds, call your cardiologist. You cannot afford to play around with this part of your daily regime.

14. You will experience some dry mouth, which is not very comfortable.

15. Do not take quick gulps of water. It is best if you sip a few ounces at a time.

16. Suck on ice cubes.

17. And lastly, although I might have mentioned this, it is a pain in the ass.

Sometimes, no matter how hard you try, you will gain water weight and you will have to take the occasional booster dose. Usually another diuretic will be used to kick the Lasix into a higher gear. I take such a drug, usually once a week. I gain an extra four or five pounds every week no matter what. I use the booster on Sundays. My wife gets out of the house while the drug is working. During the football season, this offers my wife a welcome respite.

While using the booster, I have to go every twenty minutes for about four or five hours. This is a must procedure for me. By Saturday night, I have trouble breathing and I have trouble sleeping. The booster forces the excess water off, particularly my lungs, and I feel much better.

Many CHF patients must control their fluid intake as part of their daily regime. That intake may be limited to as little as fifty ounces a day. This is not much when you consider that the bottled water companies say you should drink sixty-four ounces a day. What else would they say? They want to sell you water—you know, the stuff you can get from your tap for free.

Foods, especially fruits, provide much water so if you eat five fresh fruits and vegetables a day, the fifty ounces are adequate for your fluid requirements. Ice cream (ice cream? You have high cholesterol and you are eating ice cream?) and other frozen treats must be added as part of your fluid intake. Likewise, citrus fruit and melons, both high in water content, contribute to your daily total.

With CHF, the first place the water is going to be stored, is in your body tissue and it will be kept there and not get passed off. It is a cruel twist of fate that your body will drown itself before it will pass off the water.

Diuretics are important and useful drugs. One thing that is not often emphasized is the deleterious effect the use of diuretics has on the kidneys. It is very important you use these drugs exactly as prescribed. Your doctor will require frequent kidney and liver blood tests to ensure these drugs are causing no harm.

The next drug to be discussed is a "blood thinner." I have two artificial valves so I take this drug. Being a very lazy person, instead of making up all the language about this drug, I am stealing it directly from WebMD,[54] again.

I am including a section on warfarin. The following information was provided by Dr. Joseph Caplan (cited previously in this book). I don't know Dr. Caplan's sources but my attitude is if the doctor says this is what I need to know, than this is what I need to know. If you do take it, like me, this is information you need to know; even if you think you know it already, spend the little time it will take to read it and have your memory refreshed.

---

54   Reviewed by the doctors at The Cleveland Clinic Heart Center (2005).

Heart Disease: Warfarin and Other Blood Thinners

Warfarin, which goes by the brand name Coumadin, is an anticoagulant medication. This means that it helps prevent clots from forming in the blood. Blood thinners are used to treat some types of heart disease.

You have been prescribed warfarin because your body may be making blood clots or you may have a medical condition known to promote unwanted blood clots. It is often prescribed for patients with atrial fibrillation (an irregular heart rhythm), pulmonary embolism, and after artificial heart valve surgery or orthopedic procedures.

Blood clots can move to other parts of your body and cause serious medical problems, such as a stroke or pulmonary embolism. Warfarin will not dissolve a blood clot; however, over time, the blood clot may dissolve on its own. Warfarin may also prevent other clots from forming or prevent clots from becoming larger. You may be given other blood thinners in the hospital or even at home for a short amount of time: Heparin, Lovenox, or Fragmin. These drugs are administered either by vein (intravenous) or just under the skin into the subcutaneous fat.

Blood Testing

In order for your health care provider to determine the correct dose of warfarin, it will be necessary for you to have blood tests. The tests are performed in a laboratory, usually once a week to once a month, as directed by your doctor.

The prothrombin time (PT or Pro Time) test is used to calculate your international normalized ratio (INR). Your INR will help your health care provider determine how fast your blood is clotting and whether your medication dose needs to be changed. Illness, diet, medication changes, and physical activities may affect your INR. Tell your health care provider about changes in your health, medications (prescription and over-the-counter), or lifestyle so that appropriate dosage adjustments can be made in your warfarin therapy.

There is much you must learn when you take blood thinners. Here is another list of things you need to know:

1. Avoid getting bruised. A serious bruise can cause serious bleeding just under the skin.

2. Avoid excessive exposure to the sun.

3. Be careful using sharp instruments (you know, like not running with scissors, etc.). A little cut will bleed for a long time.

4. Use extra caution while shaving. A little nick will bleed a long time. Keep a styptic pencil handy.

5. Do not skip doses or double up if you miss a dose. However, take your regular dose if you are only a few hours late.

6. If you miss a dose for any reason, make sure you tell you INR nurse about it.

Also contact your doctor if you have any other symptoms that cause concern. Two of the most common ER visits are as a result of misuse of insulin or Coumadin. If you take either of these drugs or if you take them both, if anything suddenly gets out of kilter, do not hesitate, get immediate medical attention.

I want to make one last observation before moving on to exercise. I found myself in a conversation with a pulmonary specialist. I asked what percent of her patient load suffered not only pulmonary distress but also heart disease and obesity. The answer I found very interesting. It seems that rather a small percent of the patient load had both problems coupled with obe-sity. The reason should have been immediately obvi-ous to me but as with most things obvious and rational, I missed it.

The patient load was mostly folks over eighty years old. Patients with both pulmonary and heart disease and fifty pounds or more overweight did not usually live to be eighty years old. Patients in this category have a much higher mortality rate. Oh. Mmmm, there seems to be a message here somewhere.

Exercise

You can't get too much exercise. Exercise is not a specta-tor sport, which is exactly how most of us practice it. Most heartsick people never could qualify as being "athletic." Not with the size of that great expanse of flesh we push around in front of us and the size of the posteriors that fol-low us. I feel the need for some poetry:

Mary had a little fat burro
Its hair was brown and like fur
And everywhere that Mary went
That fat ass followed her.

Somewhere along the way to getting older and sick we got both physically and mentally lazy. Physically lazy usually presaged mentally lazy. Shame on us. We will be a burden on the next generation until our deaths. The burden will come from our neediness for care and the financial crisis we will cause on the draw down of social security and Medicare. Our children and our children's children will end up resenting us for it.

Probably the worst part of exercise is that you notice few results for quite a while once you start. As Americans, we demand immediate satisfaction. It is our God-given right to get what we need and want right now, dammit. The upshot of this attitude is that when we do not get the immediate result and the gratification that accompanies it, we quit. There must be an easier way. Say, Doc, you got a pill I can take?

There are several inhibiting factors as to how well our bodies react to exercise. Exercise is physical work. These are the only factors that matter:

- Your weight and body mass—the bigger your body the harder it is for you to move, the slower you move, and the harder it is for you to breathe. Your muscles spend more time trying to move the mass than doing any physical work you are attempting to perform.
- The percent of muscle to fat—it is twice as hard for your heart to pump blood through fat as it is to pump blood through muscle. Your muscles need oxygen and sugars to do work
- The capacity of your heart to move blood—chronic heart disease reduces the capacity of your heart to eject blood into your arteries and veins. This is called the "ejection" rate and is one of the key measurements of an echocardiogram. Further, CAD can thin the walls of your heart and this further reduces the heart's ability to get the blood flowing.
- The capacity of your lungs to get oxygen into your blood—without an adequate supply of oxygen, your muscles burn and you quickly tire. You gasp and pant.

Another inhibiting feature is we know so very little about how our bodies work. I have met very few heart patients who could or would claim to have been athletes in their early lives. Most, like me, went through periods of being fairly conscientious about exercising. I belonged to a local YMCA and played racquetball at least three times a week. And I ran my ass off. At least that is what it felt like. After more than a year of this, I was no lighter and no harder. I gave up. It was too much trouble for so little result. I thought.

Thanks to a PBS *Nova* program, I finally learned why. Here is the situation *Nova* put in place: The program selected thirteen people (volunteers) ten months before the Boston Marathon with the intent of training them all to be able to run the whole 26.2 miles. Driving 26.2 miles is a good day's effort for me. Well, not really. But the thought of physically moving my body with no aids for 26.2 miles is daunting and something I would not even attempt.

All but one of the *Nova* team finished the marathon and the lone exception was one woman suffering from shin splints who was forced to drop out several months prior to the race. The training became very rigorous in the final months leading up to the race. As a side note, tests have demonstrated that running places 110 tons of pressure on the shinbones.

The results were astounding and published in one of the prestigious medical magazines. Most importantly, the results were not at all what the sponsors anticipated prior to the experiment. Here is the first belief debunked by the experiment: exercise will cause you to lose weight. Much to everyone's surprise, this proved to be not true. Only one team member lost weight (forty-five pounds) but she had to supplement the running with strenuous aerobic training and a 1,200-calorie-a-day diet. Conclusion: exercise without dieting will not help you lose weight.

The next myth debunked was that exercise would tighten your muscles and cause you to lose clothes sizes. Not so, the experiment proved. What did happen was the nature of the exercise caused different kinds of muscle and muscle strength to be developed. Humans have muscles that are capable of differing stresses. The muscle types are two: short muscles with little staying power (these are called fast twitch muscles), which is advantageous for sprinters, and long muscles (which are called slow twitch muscles) for endurance.

The short types of muscles are what weight lifters seem to strive for, as they show good definition. Weight lifters are notorious for their inability to work for very long periods. Running creates long muscles that, although not worth a hoot for short distances, give great stamina. A fit human being can run longer and farther than dogs, antelopes, cats, and horses. A horse is the only mammal, it appears, that has endurance. Even horses with that long endurance are still no match for a human determined to run it down and eat it. Pygmies can run down elephants while the beasts are dying from the poison of their arrows. Pygmies are after that broiled elephant fat with salt and honey. There are no fat pygmies.

The 2008 Olympics gave mute proof about the types of muscles world-class athletes require. All of the endurance athletes (swimmers, runners, bikers, etc.) had long thin muscles. The athletes that required big muscles for short periods of very hard work (weight lifters, gymnasts, wrestlers, discus throwers, shot-putters, etc.) had big well-defined muscles. What is interesting is that both classes of athletes could only be described as "buff." In other words, they all looked to be in very good shape.

Another trick of evolution was to create humans with butts that change the center of balance and gravity and force us to run upright This proved essential if the human heart was to evolve to take advantage of all those muscles needed to run down and kill food. Which brings us to the next myth: the heart is stagnant in its development and once a lifestyle is created, the heart cannot be repro-grammed. Just the opposite proved to be true.

A major change all of the runners demonstrated was a new and improved pump. The way the heart worked changed entirely. It started to beat harder and improved the stroke volume. The stroke volume is the amount of blood per beat that the heart ejects and forces throughout the entire body. With each beat, the heart worked more efficiently and forced the lungs to do likewise. Think about this for just a moment...

When measured, the normal person has an "ejection fraction" of about 55 percent. This refers to the amount or volume of blood the heart, specifically the left ven-tricle chamber, is pumping with each beat. Fifty-five per-cent means the heart is emptying 55 percent of the total amount of blood in your left ventricle. It is a measure of efficiency. Patients with CAD may have lower ejec-tion fraction, especially with CHF. The lower your ejec-tion fraction the less efficient your heart is and harder time it has pumping enough blood through your body to keep you alive and feeling well. There are two ways to improve this number. One is with drugs and the other is with exercise. Sometimes a pacemaker is needed to keep your heart pumping at the right time. We will discuss the pacemaker option after completing the discussion on exercise.

OK, let's press on and I will explain what happened. It seems our heart is a wonderful organ and is just dying, or more precisely put, living, to show off what it is capable of. When faced with the challenge of doing more work, it responds, almost immediately. The runners started showing improvement in heart function in less than two weeks and they were running only a mile every other day.

Of course, if the lungs don't convert and start to work more efficiently, then all is brought to naught. Two things happened. One, the lungs responded to the pressure placed on them by the heart's increase in blood flow. Two, when the body recognized the increase in heart and lung function it sent a signal to every cell in the body ordering the myocardium, the heart muscles, and then the mitochondria, the skeletal muscles, to get busy, increase the amount of oxygen the cells would require, and suck in more sugars to nourish themselves.

Boy howdy, just think about all that happened, automatically, to make the runners' bodies more efficient machines. By the way, the mitochondria in our cells and the myocardium in our hearts are what make us different from plants. The myocardium and mitochondria are the dynamos that make us move and do work. Without mitochondria and the myocardium, we would be plants.

The last demonstrable improvement was mental in nature. The *Nova* team runners had a goal to run the entire 26.2-mile Boston Marathon route. In the end it was not just the improved physical conditioning that won the day, it was the mental toughness each of the runners developed.

There was another discovery that seemed to be somewhat of a shocker. Marathon runners do not burn huge amounts of calories. In fact, a male marathon runner is likely to burn no more than three thousand calories during the race. And it seems a woman burns fewer. Nobody knows exactly why. One thing does seem to be true. Once the body is used to an exercise level, the body will adapt to make sure the appropriate levels of sugar are stored for quick and easy use. And that storage place is not in excess hard-to-get-at fat but in the very muscles that will require the energy.

This is so important to our overall good health and well-being it bears repeating. Once the body adapts to an exercise level, the body will store energy, not as fat, but as sugars. Further, the body will store those sugars in the very muscles that will require them for work. The sad part about this is if you do not exercise, as the body has adapted to, the body will reconvert those sugars to fat and put that fat back in your butt or other unsightly places.

The diet that the runners had to adapt to was one with rich complex carbohydrates and appropriate levels of fat and sugar. Prior to the race, the runners ate small meals that were rich with foods easily converted to sugar that could be stored in THE MUSCLES and **not in fat deposits**. Gee, I said this in two paragraphs, one after the other. Must be really important to understand!

To recap, the experiment proved:

1. The heart is adaptable and will change to fill the tasks you assign it.

2. Exercise is not enough to lose weight. You must eat a good diet.

3. It is possible to change the nature of your muscles and make them work to create stamina and strength.

4. Having a goal and working diligently toward that goal creates mental toughness.

5. Eating small amounts of the right foods is more important than eating large amounts of salt, fat, and sugar-laden foods.

Information abounds about this subject and some of it is downright contradictory. For instance, the research I did on this subject stated categorically the muscles stored sugar. Well, that may not be entirely correct. *Nova Science Now* recently featured a segment about the scientist working on a new approach to fitness and weight control. He has found a drug that will trick your muscles into thinking you are exercising while you are really sitting on your butt. Wow, no pain and lots of gain. Of course, he is experimenting with mice but a mammal is a mammal.

Human beings can have one of two different kinds of muscles as stated a few pages back. The big muscles are called fast twitch muscles. Fast twitch muscles, or rather the mitochondria, feed on glucose and that is sugar. This is the reason why sugared foods can give such a quick lift in energy. Quickly used and burned sugar is just the ticket as long as short endurance exercise is occurring. This is not the way it works for the long endurance athlete.

Endurance athletes have those lean hard slow twitch muscles. The mitochondria in these muscles work an entirely different way. The mitochondria feed on fat. That's right, according to the scientist doing the work, those muscles like fat just like Jack Sprat's wife. The reason why the endurance athletes are so thin is simple: as soon as they get the fat, they use it. No passing Go to collect the $200.

This led to another observation about how all this works. Muscles that are worked on a regular basis develop more mitochondria than non-worked muscles. It is not important if the muscles are fast or slow twitch. Worked muscles have more mitochondria, and mitochondria are the energy engine that makes you work. It is a closed loop system. You work the muscles; they develop mitochondria, which require more fat to get you to move. The fat you eat is quickly used and does not appear in some unsightly place.

This fact allows us to explode another long-held myth. When muscles work, they develop more mitochondria. The development of more mitochondria is what makes for bigger muscles in the case of those seeking to develop that Mr. America build. You do not ever produce more muscle cells. Human beings have as many muscles cells as they are ever going to have when they are born.

It is not hard to see the promise of the research. Fat lazy bums like me will be able to sit on their overly large posterior and take a pill to thinness. Oh, man, isn't America great? The only drawback from my perspective is the drug will not be completely tested, proven, and approved for years. It is not even in the hands of the FDA yet and we all know how fast they work

Isn't learning fun?

This also explains something I have just not understood about myself. For the past many years I have been exercising on a rather strict basis and, as I have probably explained before, I am very lazy. I have been waiting for my muscles to begin developing. I flex a muscle and strike a pose and guess what, I still don't look like Charles Atlas. No big muscles anywhere. In fact, my muscles seem to have gotten smaller. They have not really gotten smaller, they have gotten longer. They have also gotten much harder. My exercise regime is swimming, exercise bike, and treadmill. All endurance exercises. Well, shucks, I really have been doing something right. Encouraging.

Once again, the 2008 Olympics revealed some new insights into how nutrition works. Michael Phelps, the swimmer who now owns more Olympic and world records and more gold medals than any other athlete in recorded history, requires more than ten thousand calories a day. That is almost five times more food a day than a normal person eats. However, he swims an average of five miles a day, not including his weight training. "How can anybody eat that much a day?" you may ask yourself.

I don't know. When I was working and really feeding my fat face at an alarming rate, I had days I went through almost that many calories. Well, maybe not that many, but a whole lot more than I should have. In my defense, I will say I ran through a lot of airports. Not good enough? Sorry.

Phelps consumes huge quantities of food. It is not just the food he eats that helps him get the number of calories he requires. He drinks a vitamin supplement perfected at the University of Texas. That supplement contains 2.7 grams of carbohydrates for every one gram of protein. The big brains at that school also perfected a power bar that you see the athletes munching that is the same ratio. The breakthrough came just in time for the Olympics. This ratio of carbs to protein is exactly what the athletic body requires to get the right amount of sugars into the muscles.

Our bodies are subject to all the laws of physics. A quick review of some of those laws and how they affect our bodies is in order. There is a good reason why they are called laws. The laws cannot be broken. The laws are always true, even when everything else you want to believe offers a different view. As proof, it is suggested you do the following experiment: pick up any object and drop it. Well, it fell. How 'bout that? If you do that experiment a trillion times you will get the same result.

LAW: bodies in motion tend to stay in motion. I have found that getting into a steady exercise program improves my overall ability to do more exercise. After getting used to moving for ten minutes, it becomes easy to move for fifteen minutes. Fifteen minutes quickly grows to twenty minutes, etc. You will find that a gradually increasing exercise program sort of grows on you. Interestingly enough, your mental acuity improves right along with your physical prowess.

Obverse: things at rest tend to stay at rest. Yep, once you get your posterior in that lounge chair to watch TV, it is hard to get up. The longer your posterior is attached to the chair, the harder it is to get up. Keep this up long enough, and you will become supine. Many become supine permanently.

As Dom DeLuise,[55] the comedian, used to say, "All you fat asses, get off your fat asses!" The Rules of Exercise I call "The Rules of Participation."

---

55   **Dominick "Dom" DeLuise** (August 1, 1933 – May 4, 2009) was an American actor, comedian, film director, television producer, chef, and author.

Rules of Participation

First Rule of Participation: Exercise is not easy. It requires a very special type of diligence and vigilance.

Second Rule of Participation: You must take small steps at the outset and you must find the exercise that suits your temperament. It is bad enough actually taking active steps to improve and then saddle yourself with an exercise routine you hate. Boy, I can see failure and quitting before you achieve any results if you adopt a routine you hate.

Third Rule of Participation: The best exercises for old broken-down heart patients like us are **LOW IMPACT** exercises. Applying low impact exercise will get you in the habit of doing something positive for yourself every day. As you build yourself up, you will start to see a gradual increase in the quality of your muscle tone. Some of the muscles in your body will start to get hard and we all know a hard body is a good body and a good hard body is a great body to find.

Fourth Rule of Participation: Arrange a daily exercise schedule with a start and finish time. Post the schedule on your refrigerator. On that schedule, record how much of what you did that day and also post your morning weight. It takes an awful lot of exercise to burn off the two thousand or more calories you are going to stuff into your mouth that day.

America is awash in food. An adult male with a physical job requires three thousand to thirty-five hundred calories a day. The rest of us don't really need more than two thousand to twenty-five hundred calories. And most of us really should get by on less than two thousand. Not a chance of this happening. On an average day, the 2 percent of our total population working in the food production industry (this includes everything associated with the growing, raising, manufacturing, transporting, and selling of foodstuffs) sets forth a cornucopia of forty-five hundred calories a day for every man, woman, and child. We produce more than twice as much as we could possibly eat. What happens to all those extra calories? Look behind you.

Fifth Rule of Participation: Combine low impact aerobic exercise with lightweight exercises. Why both, you may ask. The aerobic exercise will exercise your heart for stamina and help increase your ability to do work. The lightweights will improve your muscle tone. The combination will lower the amount of work the heart has to do to get blood to your muscles. This will lower your blood pressure. Your heart has to work half as hard to pump blood through muscle as it has to work to get blood through all those pounds of fat. Wait a minute, didn't I already say that? Why, I believe I did. It must be really important.

Your body does not, contrary to what the commercials claim, convert fat to muscle. Your body will burn fat as a last measure when it can find no immediately available sugar in your bloodstream. The exercise will eventually be a signal to your endocrine system to convert the fat to sugar. That is how you lose weight. The combination of a heart-smart diet and exercise will do three things: (1) increase your muscle mass and improve tone, (2) cause the body to burn off those excess pounds, and (3) lower your blood pressure and your everyday ability to do work. And (4) you will sleep better, negating the need for the sleeping pill.

Sixth Rule of Participation: Set your routine and stick with it. In short order, the routine will become second nature and your body will protest if you don't exercise. It is important you choose a routine that delivers the appropriate reward in terms of results.

Seventh Rule of Participation: Always start and end your routine with a standard set of stretching exercises. The stretching exercises at the outset of the routine will be a signal for the body to warm up and to start producing the hormones the body needs for sugar-to-energy conversions. The stretching exercises will force the release of adrenaline into your system, begin the process of increasing your heartbeat, and concentrate the lungs' transfer of oxygen to the bloodstream to oxygenate the muscles for work.

The ending stretching exercises will be a signal for the body to cool down. Over the span of the exercise period your body will release endorphins. These hormones create the sensation of well-being and happiness. Your mood will be brighter and the world will not seem like such a terrible place. The brighter mood may reduce the need for the anti-depressant medications. Your anxiety level will be toned down and you will cease to feel like you could jump out of your skin.

One last thought about low impact exercise. Our generation came up with the ridiculous idea that no pain during exercise meant no gain of benefits from exercise. If you hurt after exercising, you are doing a lot wrong. The idea of exercise is to strengthen the muscles and not hurt them. Causing harm is counterproductive to the result you are trying to achieve. You are not training to enter a weight lifting competition. You are training to lead an active healthy life.

There is an ancillary benefit of exercising and good diet. Drugs and a low activity existence cause constipation. Constipation, among its other detriments, causes you to be cranky and have headaches. A diet rich in soluble fiber from fruits and vegetables helps keep the bowels unclogged and helps pass off the toxins accumulated from the drugs. The exercise, of course, just keeps things rolling along. Regularity, while recovering from a heart procedure, is not just a requirement it is a blessing.

Although I stated at the outset of this work that the legs of the stool—diet, drug, and exercise—were listed in no particular order and all were equally important, I might have lied. Not intentionally, mind you, but through my own ignorance. I went and did some more research. Actually, I saw a program on television, either on PBS or the Discovery Channel. The program was entitled, "Living with the Caveman." That program gave me a thought about why we are the way we are.

When early people were still living in caves and out in the open, we were hunter-gatherers. We lived in relatively small groups and survived on our ability to hunt and run down game (I'll bet the animals we killed didn't think it was much of a game.) and scavenge plants and other easily reaped foods. We had to adapt the ability to eat large varieties of plants and meat. That or starve. We became omnivores and could take nutrition from almost anything. There was only one requirement: we had to stay on the move to get all that free-ranging nutrition.

Our entire body systems were adapted to be in perpetual motion. Good eyesight and stereovision in color was one of the most important adaptations. Upright stance with bodies that could run long distances was another of the more useful adaptations. But the one that may have been the most important was the ability to heal from injury, and to do it fast. We had to stay on the move so we adapted the ability to use the need for movement to help us heal. If you could not move, you quickly became bait and you became a drain on the clan. This is still true.

Exercise	Duration	Calories Expended
Watching TV	1 Hour	91
Swimming, easy	1 Hour	636
Walking, mall crawl	1 Hour	227
Walking, medium pace	1 Hour	346
Exercise bike, easy pace	1 Hour	346
Exercise bike, vigorous	1 Hour	946
Bicycling, 10–12 mph	1 Hour	546
Bicycling, 14–16 mph	1 Hour	910
Light weights, vigorous	10 Minutes	91
Stretching	10 Minutes	38
Sleeping	8 Hours	653

From the above chart, you can get an easy estimate of how many calories a day you are likely to burn during daily activity. Right at the outset, you use 653 calories just putting in your eight hours of sleep. Watching four hours of TV expends another 364 calories. See, you are making real progress at using up the 2,000 calories you are likely to eat every day. You need activity to burn only 983 more calories to balance your intake with your output. What shall you do?

You can go shopping at the mall or supermarket. At a slow pace, that pace required to look at everything, in one hour you will burn off another 227 calories; only 756 calories to go. Oops, at the mall you had a 400-calorie snack. Shucks, back up to 1,156 of needed caloric burn off.

I'm making the point this way to demonstrate how your life is now one of give-and-take at every level. If you just can't resist that piece of cake or serving of ice cream, then you will need to find a way to exercise off those calories. This is true of everything. If you want to eat more salt than the recommended amount, OK, just don't eat any for the next several days.

Now you are convinced to get off your butt and go exercise. All right, where do you go to exercise? Walking, which is a top entry for exercising, is impossible in the summer months. It is too darn hot. If you can't walk on the street, take yourself to an enclosed mall or huge air-conditioned store. When we first moved to Glendale, Arizona, we went to the Arrowhead Mall. Two times around both the top and bottom levels is about one mile. You don't have to walk fast; you just have to keep moving.

In this part of the country, due to the large numbers of senior citizens, like us, there are many places to go for exercise and aquatic exercise. Most American townships can direct you to a place for help, usually free.

The one drawback to the big mega shopping mall is all the food places. It is hard not to want to reward yourself for all the good work. The businesses in the food court know nothing goes with shopping like a quick 2,500-calorie break.

People with CAD and, in particular CHF, have another problem with exercise that needs some addressing—that is the issue of water retention. CHF patients usually take diuretics to eliminate excess water from the body, most importantly lungs. Exercise is crucial in the treatment of CHF but there is a minor conundrum. If you work too hard, you can put excess stresses on the heart, which can beget worsening heart failure, hence extra water weight, which you take off with increased doses of diuretics.

The answer is simple. You must be vigilant in exercising, and you must be extra vigilant in doing the right exercises to get in the right amount of work to stay ahead of the curve of the disease. This calls for close cooperation with your cardiologist and your physical therapist. It is just one more leg of the stool for your survival.

On the wall of the Cardiac Rehab Department of the Banner-Boswell Hospital, Sun City, Arizona, there is a sign. I am stealing it and giving it to you:

The Ten "Nevers" in Cardio Rehab

1. Never say you can't, because you'll do it anyway.
2. Never say, "It's easy," because we'll just make it harder.
3. Never say, "I want to go home." You'll just stay longer.
4. Never lose count. You will have to start over at one.
5. Never complain. No one is listening.
6. Never argue. No one cares and you'll never win.
7. Never scream or cry. That only encourages us.
8. Never look like you are enjoying it. We know how to put a stop to that.
9. Never hold your breath. If you pass out and die, we have paperwork to fill out.
10. Never lie or cheat. We know the truth and you will live to regret it.

The list is reminiscent of military basic training.

While attending a tri-weekly visit to my local cardio rehab lab, I heard another attendee lamenting the inability to lose weight. I thought back to how I managed to take off a few of the great extra poundage I was carrying around and realized I did a few things that might have been a diversion from what many dieters consider the norm. I have never been a fan of the weight loss crash diet. Here is what I did:

- Once I got into the exercise routine, I started very slowly. I was in no shape to go very fast. I started out at ten minutes a day on only two machines, exercise bike and treadmill, three times a week. Those exercise machines plus lightweights and stretching exercises. As I started to improve, I increased the length of time I was on the machines by one minute a week. I increased the weights by one pound every two weeks.

- On the dieting front, I reduced my caloric intake by two hundred calories a day. That is all. I did not try to go on a one thousand calorie-a-day regime. I would have failed. However, by making only a minor reduction a day, I started to get some slow results. Slow results are better than no results.

- Fat was a big problem. I started to add fish to my diet and more vegetables and fruits. I replaced two fatty meat meals with two fish meals. Then I replaced another two meat meals with chicken breast or turkey. Each step was incremental. No great overnight changes. Every couple of weeks I would take the next step, allow my tastes and diet to adjust and move on. It was very hard to get red meat out of my diet but over time and by taking an incremental approach, I have succeeded.

- I stopped eating butter by replacing it with olive oil. I flat out quit eating my favorite, ice cream. As Marlon Brando[56] said in the movie *Apocalypse Now*,[57] *"Oh the Horror."*

---

56 **Marlon Brando, Jr.** (April 3, 1924 – July 1, 2004), was an American actor whose body of work spanned over half a century. He is considered one of the greatest actors of all time, and was named the fourth-Greatest Male Star of All Time by the American Film Institute, and part of *Time* magazine's Time 100: The Most Important People of the Century.

57 ***Apocalypse Now*** is a 1979 American epic war film set during the Vietnam War. The plot revolves around two US Army special operations officers, one of whom, Captain Benjamin L. Willard (Martin Sheen) of MACV-SOG, is sent into the jungle to assassinate the other, the rogue and presumably insane Colonel Walter E. Kurtz (Marlon Brando) of Special Forces.

- I stopped eating candy and replaced that with an occasional piece or two of dark chocolate.
- I replaced desserts with a piece of fruit.

What you're doing right, and how to do it better[58]

So, while just futzing around on the Internet, I stumbled on this little tidbit. As you can see in the footnote, I am giving credit where credit is due. What I found so interesting in this list of thirteen signs you will live a long time is the number of the items I touch on somewhere in this work. Here is what Sandra Gordon has to say about it:

Consider this: In the twentieth century, the average life expectancy shot up thirty years—the greatest gain in five thousand years of human history. And this: centenarians—folks who make it into the triple digits—aren't such an exclusive club anymore, increasing 51 percent in number from 1990 to 2000. How to account for these dramatic leaps? Advances in health, education and disease prevention and treatments are high on the list, and that makes sense. But what you may not know is that seemingly unimportant everyday habits, or circumstances in your past, can influence how long and how well you'll live. Here, the latest research on longevity—science-based signs you're on a long-life path, plus tips on how to get on track.

Sign One: Your Mom Had You Young
If she was under age twenty-five, you're twice as likely to live to one hundred as someone born to an older mom, according to University of Chicago scientists. They suspect that younger moms' best eggs go first to fertilization, thus producing healthier offspring.

---

58 By Sandra Gordon, MSN, Health and Fitness, Women's Health, October 16, 2008

Sign Two: You're a Flourisher

About 17 percent of Americans are flourishers, says a study in *American Psychologist.* They have a positive outlook on life, a sense of purpose and community, and are healthier than "languishers"—about 10 percent of adults who don't feel good about themselves. Most of us fall somewhere in between. "We should strive to flourish, to find meaning in our lives," says Corey Keyes, PhD, a professor of sociology at Emory University. "In Sardinia and Okinawa, where people live the longest, hard work is important, but not more so than spending time with family, nurturing spirituality, and doing for others."

Sign Three: You Don't Have a Housekeeper

Just by vacuuming, mopping floors, or washing windows for a little more than an hour, the average person can burn about 285 calories, lowering risk of death by 30 percent, according to a study of 302 adults in their 70s and 80s.

Sign Four: ... and They're Healthy

If your closest friends gain weight, your chance of doing the same could increase by 57 percent, according to a study in the *New England of Journal of Medicine.* "To maintain a healthy lifestyle, it's important to associate with people who have similar goals," says Nicholas A. Christakis, MD, PhD, the study's lead researcher. Join a weight loss group, or train with a pal for a charity walk.

Sign Five: You Really Like Your Friends ...

"Good interpersonal relationships act as a buffer against stress," says Micah Sadigh, PhD, an associate professor of psychology at Cedar Crest College. Knowing you have people who support you keeps you healthy, mentally and physically: Chronic stress weakens the immune system and ages cells faster, ultimately shortening life span by 4 to 8 years, according to one study. Not just any person will do, however. "You need friends you can talk to without being judged or criticized," says Sadigh.

Sign Six: You've Been a College Freshman

A recent Harvard Medical School study found that people with more than 12 years of formal education (even if it's only one year of college) live 18 months longer than those with fewer years of schooling. Why? The more education you have, the less likely you are to smoke. In fact, only about 10 percent of adults with an undergraduate degree smoke, compared with 35 percent of those with a high school education or less, according to the CDC.

Sign Seven: You Don't Like Burgers

A few palm-size servings (about 2 1/2 ounces) of beef, pork, or lamb now and then is no big deal, but eating more than 18 ounces of red meat per week ups your risk of colorectal cancer—the third most common type, according to a major report by the American Institute for Cancer Research. Colorectal cancer risk also rises by 42 percent with every 3 1/2-ounce serving of processed meat (such as hot dogs, bacon, and deli meats) eaten per day, the report determined. Experts aren't sure why red and processed meats are so harmful, but one of their suspects is the carcinogen that can form when meat is grilled, smoked, or cured—or when preservatives, such as nitrates, are added. "You can have an occasional hot dog at a baseball game, but just don't make it a habit," says Karen Collins, RD, a nutrition advisor at AICR. And when you do grill red meat, marinate it first, keep pieces small (kebab-size), and flip them often—all of which can help prevent carcinogens from forming. If you're baking or roasting it, keep the oven temp less than 400°F.

Sign Eight: You Were a Healthy-Weight Teen

A study in the *Journal of Pediatrics* that followed 137 African Americans from birth to age 28 found that being overweight at age 14 increases your risk of developing type 2 diabetes in adulthood. Adults with diabetes are two to four times more likely to develop heart disease than those without the condition, according to the American Heart Association.

Sign Nine: You Eat Purple Food

Concord grapes, blueberries, red wine: They all get that deep, rich color from polyphenols—compounds that reduce heart disease risk and may also protect against Alzheimer's disease, according to the new research. Polyphenols help keep blood vessels and arteries flexible and healthy. "What's good for your coronary arteries is also good for your brain's blood vessels," says Robert Krikorian, PhD, director of the Cognitive Disorders Center at the University of Cincinnati. Preliminary animal studies suggest that adding dark grapes to your diet may improve brain function. What's more, in a recent human study, researchers found that eating one or more cups of blueberries every day may improve communication between brain cells, enhancing your memory.

Sign Ten: You Have Strong Legs

Lower-body strength translates into good balance, flexibility, and endurance. As you get older, those attributes are key to reducing your risk of falls and injuries—particularly hip fractures, which often quickly lead to declining health. Up to 20 percent of hip-fracture patients die within one year because of complications from the trauma. "Having weak thigh muscles is the number-one predictor of frailty in old age," says Robert Butler, MD, president of the International Longevity Center–USA in New York City. To strengthen them, target your quads with the "phantom chair" move, says

Joan Price, author of *The Anytime, Anywhere Exercise Book* (Adams, 2007). Here's how: Stand with back against wall. Slowly walk feet out and slide back down until you're in a seated position, ensuring knees aren't beyond toes and lower back is pressed against wall. Hold until your thighs tell you, "Enough!" Do this daily, increasing your hold by a few seconds each time.

Sign Eleven: You Skip Soda (Even Diet)
Scientists in Boston found that drinking one or more regular or diet colas every day doubles your risk of metabolic syndrome—a cluster of conditions, including high blood pressure, elevated insulin levels, and excess fat around the waist, that increase your chance of heart disease and diabetes. One culprit could be the additive that gives soda its caramel color, which upped the risk of metabolic syndrome in animal studies. Scientists also speculate that soda drinkers regularly expose their taste buds to natural or artificial sweeteners, conditioning themselves to prefer and crave sweeter foods, which may lead to weight gain, says Vasan S. Ramachandran, MD, a professor of medicine at Boston University School of Medicine and the study's lead researcher. Better choices: switch to tea if you need a caffeine hit. If it's fizz you're after, try sparkling water with a splash of juice. By controlling blood pressure and cholesterol levels, preventing diabetes, and not smoking, you can add six to nine and a half healthy years to your life.

Sign Twelve: You'd Rather Walk
"Fit" people—defined as those who walk for about 30 minutes a day—are more likely to live longer than those who walk less, regardless of how much body fat they have, according to a recent study of 2,603 men and women. Similarly, overweight women can improve their heart health by adding just ten minutes of activity to their daily

routine, says recent research. So take a walk on your lunch hour, do laps around the field while your kid is at soccer practice—find ways to move a little more, every day.

Sign Thirteen: You're a Tea Lover
Both green and black teas contain a concentrated dose of catechins, substances that help blood vessels relax and protect your heart. In a study of more than 40,500 Japanese men and women, those who drank five or more cups of green tea every day had the lowest risk of dying from heart disease and stroke. Other studies involving black tea showed similar results.

You really need only one or two cups of tea daily to start doing your heart some good—just make sure it's a fresh brew. Ready-to-drink teas (the kind you find in the super-market beverage section) don't offer the same health benefits. "Once water is added to tea leaves, their catechins degrade within a few days," says Jeffrey Blumberg, PhD, a professor of nutrition science and policy at Tufts University. Also, some studies show that adding milk may eliminate tea's protective effects on the cardiovascular system, so stick to just lemon or honey.

It is also important to let ALL your health care providers know you have started something like this. There may be drug-food interactions that need to be considered. There may be none known, but if you are on warfarin, they need to check to make sure your INR is not affected. And, as mentioned earlier, when the lab techs ask you if there have been any changes in your "diet" let them know about your tea adventure.[59]

(And my famous disclaimer about spelling, etc., the stuff above I copied verbatim except the last paragraph, which came from Krishna Schiller.)

At the very top of this section on exercise, it was proposed that of all the things you can do for yourself, exercise

59   Krishna Schiller as previously stated

might be the most important. No sooner had we written that than the American Heart Association[60] held a conference in New Orleans where the attendees got to hear the results of a study involving 2,231 people. All of these folks were diagnosed with <u>moderate heart failure</u> and live in the United States, Canada, and Europe. Dr. Christopher O'Connor at Duke University led the study.

The study set out to prove the benefits of exercise in the growing population of heart failure patients. In short, the test was a dismal failure. No firm link could be made between exercise and increased life span. Moreover, not only did it not prove improved life span and better survival rates, it seemed to prove the exercise would not keep those patients out of the hospital.

Dr. Harlan Krumholz, a quality-of-care researcher at Yale University, who had no role in the study, said, "Exercise is not that magic elixir that we had hoped, at least for these patients." About five million Americans have heart failure. It kills more than three hundred thousand of them and accounts for a million hospitalizations each year. Those numbers are expected to grow as the nation's population grows older.

Now here is what confuses me about all this: On one hand, the American Heart Association, as stated somewhere in this book, emphasizes the proper use and application of medicine, the importance of diet and exercise. Then in the next breath reports on the search for the "elixir" to make heart-sick patients better. Shucks, I could have saved them the time, effort, grief, and disappointment. If you don't do it all, the other two don't count.

Here are some things I learned in business:

---

60 As reported in the *Arizona Republic*, Wednesday, November 12, 2009, and written by Marilyn Marchione of the Associated Press.

- You cannot predict the results of study if you use a good methodology to conduct the study.
- If the results are something other than what you believe is intuitively correct, your intuition is incorrect.
- The raw statistics never lie. The interpretation of those statistics is open to conjecture, manipulation and misuse (in political circles this is called "spin").
- If you study the wrong thing, you get wrong results.

A Few More Important Items

There are a few open items relating to your care of CAD. We didn't know where else to address these items so we just picked this place.

Many CAD patients require pacemakers. I know I do. Pacemakers are required when the electrical system of your heart is being compromised. Medtronics,[61] a company located just outside of Minneapolis, invented the pacemaker. At least that was where they were located when I did business with them in the 1970s.

The natural electrical system sends pulses to the top, middle, and bottom of your heart. The three pulses stimulate the heart to produce the lub dub sound of the normal heart. When the system is not functioning properly, you get a flutter effect. This irregular beat is called "arrhythmia." The pacemaker smoothes out the rhythm and keeps the beat constant. Huge advances have been made in the pacemaker technology in the past thirty or so years.

61   **Medtronic, Inc.** (NYSE: MDT), based in Minneapolis, Minnesota, is the world's largest medical technology company. Listed among Fortune 500 companies, Medtronic is a publicly traded company and is listed on the New York Stock Exchange under the symbol MDT.

Once implanted, a pacemaker can last anywhere from three to six or more years. Service length is entirely dependent on use and function of the device. For instance, if your pacer is required only to smooth out occasional arrhythmic beats, the pacer will last a long time. On the other hand, if the pacer is also a defibrillator and must pace every beat of your heart, then the pacer is going to fry out in three or so years. This is no big deal. Most times replacement requires replacement of a battery.

Replacement or implantation is easy, as heart things go. I have just had my two-lead pacer replaced with a three-lead pacer. The procedure required only a one-night stay in the hospital. Most times the procedure is done as an outpatient task. It is no big deal and, unlike what you can experience with open-heart surgery, the pain is not untenable. I am a wimp (I am proud to say—I have no tolerance for pain) so I hurt and I bitched about it. Having said that, I got by and made it past the discomfort with a total of ten Tylenol 3s over a four-day period after getting out of the hospital. If I can get through it, so can you.

Pacer technology advancement continues to astound me. My newest gadget communicates to the manufacturer's headquarters. On a weekly basis, with virtually no interference from me, my pacer places a call over my house telephone line, reads the history of the activity for the past week, and transmits the data to the company's computer. If there are any anomalies, my cardiologist is notified. The old technology required me to visit the cardiologist's office every six months for a pacer check. Now that visit is required only once a year.

The last important item has to do with valve replacement. Sometimes a valve, that "spigot," wears out or breaks. The heart valve is really a simple piece of engineering. When the heart beats, the valve opens and the blood races out of the heart chamber. When the heart contracts for its next beat, the backward flow of the blood causes the valve to shut and the blood is prevented from flowing backward. Open, closed, open, closed the valve goes, depending on the rate of your pulse.

A patient faces choices when deciding on what type of valve to get. A valve recipient candidate can choose between a mechanical valve and a natural valve from a pig. The surgeon will give the candidate the options. We opted for the mechanical version. We did not think we would be having any more kids. Now I do not know what the desire to have children has to do with the selection, but it does.

A broken valve is a serious issue. I know. I have had two valves fail, the aortic valve and the mitral valve. Artificial valves have replaced both valves. My artificial valves are made of titanium and plastic. The valves are very noisy, compared to natural valves. They took some getting used to. My heart does not go lub dub. It goes click click.

Coupled with my pacemaker (I am entirely dependent on the device for a heartbeat) and the two valves, I call myself the mechanical man.

Heart Disease and Other Chronic Diseases

It is a cruel fact that many heart patients suffer from multiple chronic illnesses. Based on statistics, the order of those extra-added features would be diabetes, chronic obstructive pulmonary disease, and renal failure. In the case of a combination of heart disease and diabetes, renal failure just seems to be a freebie. Many folks have them all. I can't begin to imagine how hard a life that must be.

Faced with the fact of multiple chronic diseases, I wanted to write short sections to offer succor to those with multiple afflictions. You are not alone. There are many other chronic diseases, not the least of which are the mentally degenerative afflictions to which senior citizens are most prone. In the cases of heart disease and pick your poison, the same basic advice applies to all. We learned this from Dr. Caplan when we first started work on this book and as we mentioned in the preface and introduction.

When suffering from multiple diseases, which disease is the worst? It depends. As a layperson, my guess would be that the disease that causes you the most aggravation is the worst. Singly, none of the diseases is a day in paradise. None can be cured. All can be made livable if you adapt.

Diabetes[62]

Diabetes is the fifth-most common disease in America. This fact is not as true for the rest of the developed world but the base cause of diabetes, obesity, is on the increase. It is true here in the United States. Sixty-five percent of all diabetes deaths are from either a heart attack or a stroke. SIXTY-FIVE PERCENT! For me to write about heart disease and not write about diabetes would be criminal. I do not have diabetes but I have many family members and many friends that do and they all share one thing in common: they all have heart disease. Why? We'll get to the answer in just a moment. What appears to be true is diabetes is a lynchpin disease that dramatically affects the onset and continuation of many other chronic diseases.

It is estimated that one in every ten dollars spent on health care in this country is spent on diabetes care. This amounts to approximately $50 billion. Diabetes is big, big, big business in this country. There are more than twenty-five million diabetics. The long and the short of this means there are or will be sixteen million more people with heart

---

62   This section was written based on interviews with diabetics, nurses, dieticians, and doctors, and by researching the Web. The statistics were gleaned from the National Institutes of Health and the National Diabetes Association.

disease. The average cost per diabetes patient per year is $2,000. Ouch. This does not include the costs of the support of the other diseases with diabetes. This is just what it costs the average diabetes patient to maintain.

It does not end there. The three biggest killers and the three costliest diseases are, in order: heart disease, diabetes, and obesity. Not only do these three as a collection cause the most deaths, they account for fifty-six to fifty-nine percent of all health care dollars spent. In more ways than one, this is a very heavy burden to carry, just like all the extra poundage we carry around.

You would think that after all the years spent studying diabetes, medical science would be able to specifically explain exactly how diabetes is caused and why it works the way it does. That is certainly what I believed. I thought it would be no problem to understand the root causes and for me to give an adequate explanation. I am not concerned with the medicine of the problem. I am not a doctor. I wanted only to explain the mechanics of the disease so we could all understand it better and why, most specifically, diabetes patients almost always end up with heart disease.

In the past couple of years, as we were writing this book, I had occasion to speak with many sufferers. I, in an effort to learn how their lives were affected, asked a lot of questions. I made a real pain of myself. I am sorry for that. However, I learned a really important fact: most, if not all, accepted the link between diabetes and heart disease, as if it were some curse that could not be avoided. Hmmmmm. There is something wrong with the logic here.

My conclusion was this: If a patient suffers from diabetes, and has suffered for some time, and is diagnosed with heart disease, it is accepted as just a fait accompli and is just one more doctor to see in a never-ending cycle of doctor visits. It is just some more medicine to take. In my opinion, this is just stinking thinking. Worse, the patients so accept this fact they do little or nothing to learn why the two diseases go hand in hand. Doctors, being so busy, cannot take the time to educate. We explained why in the section on how doctors are compensated.

I was able to learn, without too much trouble, those who are most at risk of getting diabetes. I found this most informative, as it seems those most likely to get diabetes are also most likely to get CAD. (This is an acronym we have not used for a while. In case you forgot, it means coronary artery disease.) Anyone can develop diabetes, but some people are more at risk than others. You are at greater risk for diabetes if you (items underlined mean those items are the major contributing factors to other chronic diseases):

- Are over forty-five years old.
- Are overweight.
- Are African American, Hispanic/Latino, Asian, Pacific Islander, or American Indian.
- Have a family history of diabetes.
- Have high cholesterol.
- Have had gestational diabetes during pregnancy.
- Have given birth to a baby that weighed more than nine pounds.
- Exercise fewer than three times a week.

The sad truth is the longer a patient suffers from diabetes, the better the chance the patient has of developing heart disease. This is true for both type 1 and type 2 diabetes. It appears it cannot be avoided.

The three ethnic groups that are seeing the fastest and largest growth of their populations developing diabetes are Native Americans, Mexican Americans, and African Americans. Guess what, these three groups are also experiencing the fastest increase of heart disease. The same reason for this increase in these populations is change of diet. There are two mitigating circumstances.

One circumstance is the change of diet as a result of an increased standard of living or, more properly stated, increased income. The increased income permits money to be spent on more foods that are processed and contain large quantities of processed flour, processed sugars, trans fat, and salt. These are fast foods and salty, fatty snack foods. Pass the potato chips, please. Say, how 'bout some more of those nachos with extra cheese? Thank you. Twinkie, anyone?

The other circumstance is counterintuitive and the opposite is true. Fast food, high in fructose corn syrup is far cheaper than healthy non-process fruits veggies, and lean meat. That is why the urban poor disproportionately suffer from obesity and heart disease

The subgroup that is exhibiting the greatest increase within these populations is children. Money not only makes the world go around, it makes the kids round. But then, why should minorities be excluded from all the wealth and fatness? American kids in general are the fattest they have ever been in our history. The burden they will place on the health care system will be staggering. Ooops, sorry, I got off on a tangent there for a moment. But, as a point of interest, what do your kids and grandkids look like?

This situation of ever-fattening kids is on the verge of being pandemic. Doctors, pediatricians, in fact, are finding themselves having to prescribe drugs to lower cholesterol in young children. Now, "ain't that a revoltin' development." Kids, less than twelve years old, having not even gone through puberty, are contracting adult chronic diseases. Not only are pediatricians prescribing insulin and anti-cholesterol drugs, but hypertension drugs as well. It may look like a kid, act like a kid, think like a kid, but it eats like an adult and now has adult diseases.

The cause of diabetes is the inability of the pancreas to make enough insulin to keep high levels of sugar out of your blood stream. Not only does it not properly process sugars, it appears the failure extends to how the body will process fats. From your reading so far, you can see where this is going, can't you? You have already learned the body transforms fats into sugar to be stored in the muscles for immediate work or it transforms sugar into fat that it stores in the fat deposits being saved for times of emergency that never come.

(It appears that I may not have that exactly correct. One of the vetting docs says what I really want to say is this: This is only true for Type 1 diabetes that represents about 5% of all diabetes. 95% of diabetes is Type 2 diabetes, 'adult onset diabetes' though it is now a disease of childhood due to overweight and obesity. The cause for Type 2 diabetes (95% of the time) is insulin resistance that is due to overweight and obesity. It is not about the pancreas. The incidence of Type 2 diabetes has doubled in the past 10 years in America because of the obesity epidemic. The treatment for diabetes is not controlling blood sugar but weight loss. The vast majority of Type 2 diabetics are rid of their diabetes and medications when they lose weight and approach or reach a healthy BMI of 24.)[63]

The fat it has most trouble with is the worst type, which is LDL. The body has a very hard time of passing LDL fats off. The only two ways to help the body get rid of the LDL fat is to either take drugs specifically designed to move the fat out or increase the amount of HDL fat you eat. The HDL fats actually escort the LDL fat out of the body. We talked about this in fairly great detail earlier in the book. For diabetics, this is even more important.

You might think about the relationship between LDL and HDL in terms of dating. When an HDL sees an LDL it

63 Dr. Mark Nelson, cardiologist, internist and obesity specialist.

says, "Hey, baby, whatcha doin'?" The LDL replies it has no pressing engagements. "I'm just laying around gumming up the works." The HDL says, "Let's blow this pop stand. But while we are at it, I can take your friend along for the ride." Wherein the HDL escorts two LDLs to the liver and out of the body for the price of one. (Sounds a little like carload night at the drive-in movie.) This becomes even more important when we get to renal failure.

Fat to sugar, sugar to fat is the way the fats go round in the body. By reducing the overall amount of fat, and specifically the LDL fats, the less the pancreas has to process and the less strain on an already-failing organ. Less fat equals less sugar. High sugar levels mean high glucose levels and that is the danger. Sugars, in general, and processed or corn sugars in particular, are really bad news and combined with high levels of LDL produce the double whammy diabetics have to learn to live without.

Over time, high blood glucose levels damage nerves and blood vessels, leading to complications such as heart disease and stroke, the leading causes of death among people with diabetes. Uncontrolled diabetes can eventually lead to other health problems as well, such as vision loss, kidney failure, and amputations. We will address the issue of renal failure in just a bit.

It is not the usual case, but heart disease patients can also develop diabetes. It is usually the other way around. However, a heart patient does need to look for a set of newly developing symptoms. Diabetes often has no symptoms or warning signs. The only way to be sure is to have your blood tested for glucose (blood sugar). If symptoms do appear, they might include:

- Feeling tired
- Feeling irritable
- Urinating more than normal
- Being very thirsty

- Being very hungry
- Unexplained weight loss
- Blurred vision

If you are experiencing some of these symptoms or think that you might be at risk for diabetes, be sure to talk to your doctor about getting tested. This is important. You may develop some of these symptoms and chalk them up to the drugs you are taking, your perceived generally deteriorating condition from the heart disease, or general ignorance and stupidity. Just because you don't feel well, does not mean your heart is the problem.

Diabetes can lead to heart and blood vessel disease. Got that? Here's what else:

- Heart disease strikes people with diabetes twice as often as people without diabetes.
- In people with diabetes, cardiovascular complications occur at an earlier age and often result in **premature death**.
- People with diabetes are two to four times more likely to suffer strokes and, once having had a stroke, are two to four times as likely to have a recurrence.

Dr. Darry Johnson, a neurologist, pointed out to me that atherosclerosis is the same wherever it strikes. In other words, the causes of heart attacks are the same causes of strokes. The link is inescapable. What is interesting is that all the risks fall under a relatively new diagnosis: metabolic syndrome. What follows is from the National Institutes of Health.

What Is Metabolic Syndrome?

Metabolic syndrome: Suddenly, it's a health condition that everyone's talking about. While it was identified less than twenty years ago, metabolic syndrome is as widespread as pimples and the common cold. According to the American Heart Association, forty-seven million Americans have it. That's a staggering almost one out of every six people.

Indeed, metabolic syndrome seems to be a condition that many people have, but no one knows very much about. It's also debated by the experts—not all doctors agree that metabolic syndrome should be viewed as a distinct condition.

So what is this mysterious syndrome—that also goes by the scary-sounding name Syndrome X—and should you be worried about it?

Understanding Metabolic Syndrome

Metabolic syndrome is not a disease in itself. Instead, it's a group of risk factors—high blood pressure, high blood sugar, unhealthy cholesterol levels, and abdominal fat.

Obviously, having any one of these risk factors isn't good. But when they're combined, they set the stage for grave problems. These risk factors double your risk of blood vessel and heart disease, which can lead to heart attacks and strokes. They increase your risk of diabetes by five times.

Metabolic syndrome is also becoming more common. But the good news is that it can be controlled, largely with changes to your lifestyle.

Risk Factors for Metabolic Syndrome

According to the American Heart Association and the National Heart, Lung, and Blood Institute, five risk factors make up metabolic syndrome.

Large Waist Size	*For men:* 40 inches or larger *For women:* 35 inches or larger
Cholesterol: High Triglycerides	*Either* 150 mg/dL or higher or using a cholesterol medicine
Cholesterol: Low Good Cholesterol (HDL)	*Either* *For men:* less than 40 mg/dL *For women:* less than 50 mg/dL or using a cholesterol medicine
High Blood Pressure	*Either* Having blood pressure of 130/85 mm Hg or greater or using a high blood pressure medicine
Blood Sugar: High Fasting Glucose Level	100 mg/dL or higher

To be diagnosed with metabolic syndrome, you would have at least *three* of these risk factors. What is surprising to me is the number of people I see walking around that probably have all five of the factors. Yet they are not diagnosed with any disease. As comedian Lewis Black says, "They (the docs) just don't know. What can be safely stated is this: If they ain't got it now, they will...or they get hit by a truck."

As stated when we began this particular discussion, I am interested in the mechanics of the disease and why it would have such devastating effects on so many other things. Nobody could explain exactly how it works. The professional folks could explain only the observable circumstances like the five listed things above. They could not explain the steps of effect. I had to work it out for myself and, being free from actual medical knowledge and preconceived ideas of how stuff works, here is my conclusion:

1. The pancreas produces insulin.

2. The insulin is the hormone that facilitates the movement of sugars (glucose) into the body's cells. It is the only substance that is the osmosis catalyst to move the sugars. Remember this.

3. When the pancreas fails (for whatever reason and there are many), the ability to produce insulin is restricted. The failure to produce enough insulin is the only cause of diabetes.

4. Every organ, cell, muscle, and you name it, needs sugar to work and maintain. Everything, everything.

5. The diabetic pancreas does not produce adequate insulin.

6. Inadequate insulin makes it impossible to pass adequate sugar and fat to everything, everything.

7. Not enough sugar and fat, inadequate cell function, and cell deterioration.

8. Cell deterioration causes the onset of other disease.
9. Heart and cardio vascular disease will quietly and inevitably ensue.
10. Sixty-five percent of those so afflicted will die.
11. Bad odds.
12. I am willing to make a small wager that it is just this simple. But then, I am not a doctor.

CAD patients with diabetes suffer something else. Worse, they don't even know it is happening when it occurs. They are at increased risk for a "silent" heart attack. Patients that have had silent heart attacks don't even know they have had them. They don't hurt. Do you remember when I mentioned my cardiologist wanting me to emphasize that the severity of the pain is not an indicator of the severity of the heart attack? Well, this is why. The pain of a silent heart attack will not make you sit up in bed or fall over grasping your chest. It is the other symptoms, the ones you ignore because there is no pain, that are the killers.

Long periods of time may elapse before a patient is ever diagnosed as having had a silent heart attack. It is from other tests the problem is discovered. What may be a routine EKG can discover the past event. The heart attack will have killed some heart tissue and the EKG will show the damage. Or an echocardiogram will highlight the problem. Or any number of other tests will reveal the extent of the damage. Only one thing is true about all the tests that will have revealed the history: it is too late to undo the problem.

If you are diabetic and suddenly start to sweat, get sick to your stomach, suffer any numbness to your left arm or jaw, have a sudden headache and don't know why, and experience any of the other symptoms of heart attack listed previously, do not delay. Get yourself to the emergency room. You can be having the onset of either a silent heart attack or stroke. Don't be macho or a martyr. The life you might destroy is not just your own. A blood test looking for a certain set of hormones present only when a heart attack is occurring will confirm the diagnosis.

About the first advice given to a newly diagnosed diabetic is dietary. A low carb diet restricting sugars is the best deal. In fact, diabetics are told to get on a heart-healthy diet. I am sure that if you are diabetic you have been told to get on a heart-healthy diet. The approaches advocated in the book for living with heart disease are very similar for those living with diabetes.

Testing is the other big deal of maintenance for a diabetic. Heart patients are not burdened with a particularly onerous testing regime. Not so for diabetes patients. Testing for blood sugar levels is a many-times-a-day task that may not be put off or neglected. Sugar is not the only thing to worry about. By neglecting the sugar level testing, the body has to cope with ongoing out-of-bounds situations.

The onset of the other chronic diseases is a slow and inevitable process. Compare it to a minor sore. I had a friend in the service many years ago. He told the story of an ingrown fingernail or hangnail. The darn thing would never heal. Instead, it got worse and worse, no matter what he did. The usual fingernail biting did not fix the problem. It eventually got so bad, he was faced with the possibility of amputation of the finger. This proves a basic law of physics: left to themselves, things only get worse. Ignoring the testing and just letting things get by only makes matters far worse.

It also reminds me of the great Joe Louis.[64] Joe was scheduled to box one of the many "bums of the month" during his career. Joe's opponent bragged he was not worried about Joe's punch. "I am going to run around the ring so he will never get a chance to hit me." Joe thought

---

64 **Joseph Louis Barrow** (May 13, 1914–April 12, 1981), better known as **Joe Louis**, was the world heavyweight boxing champion from 1937 to 1949.

about it for a moment and then replied, "He can run but he can't hide." You can run away from the testing, but you can't hide from the disease.

The National Institutes of Health has issued some guidelines for patients with both diabetes and heart disease:

People with diabetes can take some steps to lower their risk of heart disease and stroke. Learn the diabetes **ABCs.** Target ranges are as follows:

A A1C < 7 percent. Check at least twice a year.
B Blood Pressure < 130/80 mmHg. Check at every doctor's visit. (I don't know about this. I would think that blood pressure of 120/80 would be far more desirable.)
C Cholesterol-LDL < 100 mg/dl. Check at least once a year.

Patient education is critical. People with diabetes can reduce their risk for complications if they are educated about their disease, learn and practice the skills necessary to better control their blood glucose, blood pressure, and cholesterol levels, and receive regular checkups from their health care team.

Lifestyle changes are extremely valuable. Smokers should stop smoking and overweight men and women with diabetes should develop a moderate exercise regimen under the guidance of a health care provider to help them achieve a healthy weight. (Could this get any wimpier? Should stop smoking? Hey, moron, if you have diabetes and you smoke, well, you know what I think about that.)

Health care team education is vital. Because people with diabetes have a multi-system chronic disease, they are best monitored and managed by highly skilled health care professionals trained with the latest information on diabetes to help ensure early detection and appropriate treatment of the serious complications of the disease. A team approach to treating and monitoring this disease serves the best interests of the patient.

Caregiver notes: Huh? What is needed is active participation on the part of the caregiver to ensure your patient does all the right things. Highly skilled health care professionals are not coming into your home and monitoring what your patient eats, how and if your patient exercises, and how and when the appropriate testing is done. Professionals are paid for a Level One Service. That is fifteen minutes a visit. Who are you gonna call for the day-to-day interventions and support that are really needed? Dr. Phil does not make house calls. Nor does Dr. Oz.

Where is the advice about exercise? What's going on here? A moderate exercise program? Get off your fat, sick, heart disease, diabetic ass and get moving. Drop that Twinkie, those nachos, and that soda.
Four things:

1. Exercise
2. Diet
3. Medicine
4. Testing

Tattoo them on the inside of your eyelids.

Diabetes is not curable, but it is reversible and remedial. It is also possible to alleviate the other chronic diseases. Most importantly, it is manageable. But you cannot take a passive role in the management of your disease. Oh, and don't forget, any changes in how you feel or changes in medications require you to notify every doctor you see, immediately.

Chronic Obstructive Pulmonary Disease (COPD)[65]

Based on appearance, you can't tell a person suffering from COPD. In fact, they might even look pretty healthy. The sufferer might appear to be trim and fit. With severe COPD there is shortness of breath. The shortness of breath greatly limits activity, in short the ability to exercise. The loss of the ability to exercise causes the deconditioning of the muscle mass. In severe and more advanced COPD, the lungs' ability to deliver oxygen is impaired. Exercise becomes harder and harder with the progression of the lung disease. Pulmonary disease can progress very slowly so the decline is not immediately noticeable. Muscle mass that does not get enough exercise will atrophy and become flaccid and flabby. The muscle mass shrinks in size and the patient appears to be trim. Obese patients suffering from COPD run additional risks. Wait, it gets worse.

Now add to this the heart's inability to function properly in patients suffering from more chronic forms of coronary artery disease. The heart, charged with pumping to the muscles and already impaired, does not even have properly oxygenated blood to pump. All this does not happen overnight. There is, in fact, a disorderly progression.

Many times, the first symptom of both heart disease and COPD is shortness of breath. You might know the feeling. It becomes harder to do simple things like walk long distances from the parking space to the mall or climb steps; you start to feel like you are mountain climbing. You find yourself panting. Your first stop will probably be to a primary care giver, who will put you through the testing cycle. (See page 26–27.)

The primary care provider, trying to treat shortness of breath, and finding no indication of heart disease, will more often than not send you to the pulmonary specialist.

---

65   This section would not have been written without the guidance and support of Dr. Shannon Valenzuela.

This is a good thing. The pulmonary doc will be looking for shortness of breath from any of these causes of pulmonary disease:

- Pulmonary disease, which includes a list of diseases, that is beyond our purview.
- Anemia – It never occurred to me that anemia could cause shortness of breath.
- Cardiac
- Deconditioning – Morbidly obese.
- Thromboembolic disease – Blood clots that have traveled to lungs.

Obviously four of the above are really not germane to our discussion.

(Most PCPs are well trained in COPD and will complete the work-up appropriately. Odd cases or cases not responding to evidence-based therapies may be referred to Pulmonologists.[66])

Earlier in the book we made mention of the impact of body fat on the ability to breathe. Having a very big belly seriously impairs the ability of the lungs to expand fully. It is a simple problem of mechanics. Your lungs must fully expand and contract; to do that, they need space. With normal amounts of body fat, the diaphragm contracts down into the abdominal cavity. This is the lungs' normal and necessary expansion inside the chest cavity that causes so much pain after open-heart surgery.

The amount of space the lungs have to expand is finite. Your body is not going to grow any more space. There is just so much stuff your body has planned to put into its available space and fat is not one of the things that make up the stuff. The body has to hide the fat—fat chance. The fat encroaches into the areas reserved for important things like

---

66 Dr. Mark Moeller, M.D. Family Practice, Sutter West Medical Group, Davis, Ca.

organs and muscles. As this encroachment occurs, less and less space is available for the lungs. In other words, there is no place for the lungs to go to expand.

Lung expansion is limited, the amount of work the lungs are capable of doing is limited, in some cases oxygen delivery is impaired, the amount of work the muscles is capable of doing is limited, and your ability to move is limited. Most importantly, your ability to survive is limited. Say, how about another cheeseburger to go with that wheeze? Think of cheese fries as wheeze fries.

Your body can be compared to an internal combustion engine with the lungs supplying the air to make the spark plugs (muscles) fire (energy and motion). To keep this chain of events working smoothly, a few basic steps are required. Here they are:

- The very first one for both cardiac and pulmonary disease is (and this should come as no surprise) NO SMOKING. Gee, who would have thought this is the most important of all?
  · Doctors tell me that patients who do not give up the weed will give up the ghost. Worse, those patients that smoke will break down and cry and lament how hard it is to quit smoking. I say this to all those who continue to smoke after being diagnosed with either or both cardiac and pulmonary disease: Up yours. Go someplace far away from me and smoke yourself to death; the sooner the better.
- It is imperative to establish and maintain good communication among all your doctors. As a patient, you may not remain passive on this point. You would not be out of line if you asked to see the records that the docs are passing among themselves. Knowledge is power.

- *Caregiver notes: As the caregiver, you must be up to date on all that is going on. Remember, you are the captain of the team.*
- When anything changes, especially if it changes for the worse, more or different therapy might be in order. All of your docs must know of the changes.
- Both the pulmonary specialist and the cardiologist must be in complete sync when any surgery is required.
- Surgery puts a co-sufferer at greater risk. Those risks must be thoroughly discussed with both docs. Also, see statement above about smoking.
- Learn to love and use the incentive spirometer.
- It is imperative that your pain be appropriately treated. Poorly or mistreated pain can and does lead to a host of side complications, not limited to but including stress, depression, and anxiety (all of which will be discussed in great detail later in the book).
- Colds are nothing to sneeze at (I just could not resist). Colds have a nasty habit of settling in the chest. Lack of mobility can lead to pneumonia. Pneumonia for sufferers of both pulmonary and cardiac disease is really bad news.

Drugs are a big part of daily life. In an earlier section, we dealt with the importance of living with medications. With both diseases, some extra precautions are in order:

- Take care to ensure there is no adverse reaction between drugs taken for different diseases. Ask your doctors what those drugs are, and when new drugs are being prescribed do

not be afraid to speak up and challenge your docs about side effects.
- *Caregiver notes: If your patient does not do this, you should.*
- Some pulmonary drugs can affect cardiac disease, most notably broncho dilators that can stimulate your heart rate.
- Some cardiac drugs can cause pulmonary problems. Amiodarone, an arrhythmia drug, can cause problems. Likewise, beta-blockers for asthma patients cause problems.
- Over-the-counter drugs must be taken with care and if you have any questions you must immediately ask your doctors.
- At every visit with your doctor, review your entire medication regime.

Cardiac disease and pulmonary disease make life a hassle on a massive scale. However, having said that, the fact of the matter is this: You can live a long time with both. And your life can be productive, fulfilling, and worthwhile. All you have to do is adopt the lessons taught in this book and adapt to the new lifestyle.

Renal Failure[67]

Well, here it is. This is the ultimate end game chronic disease. This disease is such a horror I have put it off for as long as I could. Chronic kidney disease (chronic renal failure) is the long-standing, progressive deterioration of renal function. Symptoms develop slowly and include anorexia,

---

67   This section was written after extensive research on many Web sites and interviews with health care professionals. The most important Web sites were the American Heart Association, The National Kidney Fund, Merck On Line Manuals for Health Care Professionals, and, of course, that old standby, WebMD.

nausea, vomiting, stomatitis, dysgeusia, nocturia, lassitude, fatigue, pruritus, decreased mental acuity, muscle twitches and cramps, water retention, undernutrition, GI ulceration and bleeding, peripheral neuropathies, and seizures. In the footnote, I explain where I got all this stuff. Frankly, I don't understand the medical terms. I do understand how those symptoms effect and affect heart disease and vice versa.

It is possible to live with renal disease for a very long time since, as the paragraph above says, it is a long-standing progressive disease. But to cut to the chase, it is devastating and will eventually get to end stage renal disease (ESRD). I quote the American Heart Association:

Diabetes mellitus is the primary cause of ESRD. Diabetic renal disease (diabetic nephropathy) represents a long-term complication of diabetes that results from direct vascular abnormalities. One of the early renal manifestations of diabetes is the presence of small quantities of albumin in the urine (microalbuminuria), which is an early sign of kidney disease. Susceptible individuals eventually develop persistent proteinuria, which presents increased risks of developing progressive renal disease and of death due to chronic vascular disease (CVD). Hence, the vascular abnormalities accompanying diabetes can produce chronic renal disease which, in turn, increases the risk for CVD. This scenario illustrates the intimate interaction between the kidney and CVD: **Kidney disease can represent either a cause or a consequence of CVD.**

Here is what it all boils down to: heart disease can bring on renal failure, for a variety of reasons, only some of which we will talk about; vice versa, renal failure can bring on serious heart disease that will lead to death. To understand why, it is necessary to have an idea as to just what the kidneys do. They are a marvel of engineering and the ultimate filtration system.

Think of your kidneys like a pasta strainer or filter. Your kidneys keep some things in your body that you need, and get rid of other things that you don't. The kidneys also do many other jobs that you need to live. Your kidneys:

- Make urine
- Control fluid levels
- Remove wastes and extra fluid from your blood
- Control your body's chemical balance
- Help control your blood pressure
- Help keep your bones healthy
- Help you make red blood cells

The real trick the kidneys do is keeping your chemical system in balance. Almost everything you put into your body, in high enough quantities, can be toxic. The three main minerals your body depends on to control the entire electrolyte system are sodium, potassium, and calcium. A host of other minerals exist, including phosphorus and zinc, that play minor parts in keeping the systems function but those three are the key players. When this function gets out of whack, the primary victim is the heart.

When there is too little of the minerals in the blood system, the electrolyte system malfunctions. When there is too much, your system malfunctions. Just like what was best for Baby Bear, the kidneys keep everything just right.

Hypertension is a cause of kidney disease. Heart patients usually have hypertension. By definition, this puts heart patients at risk. Anyone can get chronic kidney disease at any age. However, some people are more likely than others to develop kidney disease. You may have an increased risk for kidney disease if you:

- Have diabetes.
- Have high blood pressure.
- Have a family history of chronic kidney disease.

- Are older.
- Belong to a population group that has a high rate of diabetes or high blood pressure, such as African Americans, Hispanic Americans, Asian, Pacific Islanders, and American Indians.

Say, that list looks suspiciously familiar. Do you sense a developing pattern here? The pattern gets even clearer when considering the symptoms of chronic kidney disease. Most people may not have any severe symptoms until their kidney disease is advanced. However, you may notice that you:

- Feel more tired and have less energy
- Have trouble concentrating
- Have a poor appetite
- Have trouble sleeping
- Have muscle cramping at night
- Have swollen feet and ankles
- Have puffiness around your eyes, especially in the morning
- Have dry, itchy skin
- Need to urinate more often, especially at night

A cardiac patient may ignore these symptoms and attribute them to his or her heart disease. Bad on you if you do. Heart disease can cause kidney disease and vice versa. I know I have already written this but it is very important. This fact is a main reason why your cardiologist does so much blood testing.

Your kidneys play a role in getting toxins out of your blood. To accomplish this it filters every drop of your blood every hour, twenty-four hours a day with no time off for vacations or good behavior. If your kidneys call in sick, the whole plant shuts down. Talk about a critical employee.

You know all those drugs you take to stay well? Yep, they are all toxic. The kidneys have to get that stuff out of your body and they don't like it. It is a dirty job but somebody has to do it. Urea, the end stage product of protein metabolism, is produced in the liver (just what we needed, another organ affected by kidney failure) and is excreted by the kidneys. Urea is formed from amino acids and ammonia compounds and it is this substance that gives urine its undesirable aroma. However, that smell tells you that things are working as required. It also accounts for the color. When either the smell or color is something other than what is expected, that is trouble and you must tell your doctor.

While doing all that filtering, the kidneys continually evaluate just how much fluid you have on board. Your body needs only so much fluid and anything other than that is just too darn much. The result of having too much fluid on board is well known to all; say, just where is the restroom? The kidneys will automatically adjust the concentration of your urine, which is why urine loses its yellow color when expelling excessive fluids.

As if the function of filtration is not enough, the kidneys do a few more things of great importance including regulate blood pressure, make red blood cells, and promote strong bones.

Treatment[68]

We are going to jump right to treatment for a moment. It is a bit out of order but it is necessary to discuss this subject to make other important points. Treatment includes the following:

---

68   Merck On Line Medical Manuals for Health Care Professionals

- Control of underlying disorders. (Kidney disease is linked to so many other chronic conditions, a holistic view of treatment must be taken.)
- Possible restriction of dietary protein, phosphate, potassium.
- Vitamin D supplements.
- Treatment of anemia and heart failure.
- Doses of all drugs adjusted as needed.
- Dialysis for severely decreased GFR, uremic symptoms, or sometimes hyperkalemia or heart failure.

Underlying disorders and contributory factors must be controlled. In particular, controlling hyperglycemia in patients with diabetic nephropathy and controlling hypertension in all patients substantially slows deterioration of GFR.

Potassium intake is closely related to meat, vegetable, and fruit ingestion and usually does not require adjustment. However, foods (especially salt substitutes) rich in potassium should generally be avoided.

This information was gleaned from Merck as noted in the footnote. Merck leaves out exercise. I wonder why?

Chronic Diseases – The Bigger Picture

When my cardiologist, Dr. Caplan, first taught me the treatment for four chronic diseases was very similar and the everyday advice for living for them all the same, I just took that at face value. After all, what did I know? It never occurred to me there was a much bigger picture of the problem of cardiac disease. I just went along with the program. "I vas yust following orders." This is not something you would be likely to ever hear me say.

Consider the inexorable chains of events among all the organs involved.

1. The heart pumps blood containing glucose and oxygen to the organs, muscles, and everything, everything. The blood carries off the waste from the everything, everything for disposal and removal from the body.

2. The pancreas produces insulin, which is the facilitator of moving glucose into the muscles, organs, and everything, everything so everything, everything can work.

3. The lungs dissolve oxygen into the bloodstream and extract carbon dioxide from the bloodstream.

4. The blood is the carrier and delivers nutrients and oxygen in and waste and carbon dioxide out. The most essential fluid the kidney will monitor the level of is blood.

5. The kidneys filter the blood and remove the wastes. During the filtration process, the kidneys monitor the chemical levels in the blood and monitor the fluid levels. If the fluid levels are too low, the kidneys make you thirsty. If too high, the excess fluid is passed to the bladder. If the nutrient levels in the blood get low, the kidneys send a signal to make you hungry.

6. During the filtration process, the kidneys validate the red blood cell level. Since the red blood cells are the specific carriers of all the required goodies, if the cell count starts to get low, the kidneys send the message to the bone marrow to produce more red cells.

7. While all this is going on the kidneys continually monitor the blood pressure trying to prevent hypertension.

8. As long as all this functions properly, your life merry-go-round keeps going around. When the systems break down, your nice comfortable merry-go-round turns into a roller coaster.

The results of this chain ensure your ability to get one foot in front of the other and to move forward. Step by step. If the chain malfunctions the following ensue:

1. If the pancreas produces too little insulin, you get tired, hungry, and thirsty. You can no longer move forward.

2. If the lungs don't dissolve enough oxygen into the blood, you get tired. You can no longer move forward.

3. If the heart function is impaired, nothing gets to the cells and you can no longer move forward.

4. If the kidney function is crippled, the blood is not filtered, your electrolyte system crashes, your heart and other organs cannot function, and you cannot move forward. Or in any other direction.

5. If you cannot move forward, you cannot move at all and this is called death.

Gee, that's not so complicated at all. In fact, presented like that, it's pretty simple.

If you have read this before, don't stop me. Here is how you beat the system:

1. Test, test, test
2. Diet
3. Proper medications taken the proper way
4. Exercise, exercise, exercise

I'll bet this is all starting to sound familiar.

Dental Care

You might consider it strange to talk about dental care in a free-ranging discussion about heart disease. Not only is it not strange, it is mandatory, although oftentimes over-looked by the internists and cardiologists caring for you. Good dental care is very important. The reason is simple. There is a direct line from your heart to your jaw and brain. It is the carotid artery. From heart to jaw and brain, do not pass go but do stop and pick up the money.

An infection caused by dental disease is offered a clear path to infect the entire body. An infection is a serious issue for a CAD patient and even more important if you must take Coumadin. Another sad fact of aging is the decline in health of the teeth. The teeth start to wear out and crumble. The dental woes may, at the outset, be painless. However, if not immediately treated, they could cause far worse problems than a toothache. Brush your teeth twice a day and floss. And get your teeth examined and cleaned on a regular basis.

Depression and Stress[69]

Boys and girls, it is now time to talk about the worst part of the whole damn ordeal: depression and the accompany-

---

69 This section was written with the help of Dr. Michael Cofield, Psychologist, and Mary Ann Zimmerman, Therapist.

ing stress and anxiety. In your experience, you will probably find nobody prepares you for the depression that is associated with serious coronary procedures. Here is what you need to know about depression:

- Depression is the leading cause of disability in the United States.[70]
- Depression is now the leading cause of disability in the world.[71]
- Chronic illness increases one's chance for depression.[72]
- Depression is treatable and most people who are treated show improvement.[73]

Heart disease is a most serious chronic illness.

Caregiver notes: Nobody tells you about this aspect of serious heart disease. Of all the things you as a caregiver will have to cope with, this is the worst. Although often mental in appearance, you must remember the depression is being caused by a mixture of the medications, circumstances and behavioral factors. You need to keep reminding yourself this is the case.

---

70 US Department of Health and Human Services. Mental Health: A Report of the Surgeon General Executive Summary. Rockville, MD: US Department of Health and Human Services, Substance Abuse and Mental Health Services Administration, Center for Mental Health Services, National Institutes of Health, National Institute of Mental Health, 1999.

71 World Health Organization Web site. The World Health Report 2001/Mental Health: New Understanding, New Hope. [Message from the Director-General]. Retrieved from www.who.int/ whr/2001/dj_message/en.

72 US Department of Health and Human Services. Fact Sheet: Depression Co-Occurring with General Medical Disorders. Bethesda, MD. National Institutes of Health, National Institute of Mental Health, 1999.

73 US Department of Health and Human Services. Fact Sheet: Depression Co-Occurring with General Medical Disorders. Bethesda, MD. National Institutes of Health, National Institute of Mental Health, 1999.

Many years ago, John Chancellor,[74] then the evening news anchor for NBC, required bypass surgery. As could be expected, given the state of the art at that time, the surgery was an emergency. John went from the stress EKG test to the operating room. You may have had the same experience so you know how frightened John was. Fortunately, for John, the test was being done at Johns Hopkins University Hospital.[75] No ambulance was required; the medics just wheeled him into the cardiac OR.

Johnny Carson[76] was interviewing Chancellor on Carson's show, just prior to Chancellor returning to work. During the interview, Chancellor recounted how the aftermath of the surgery was worse than the surgery itself. Chancellor said the post-surgery time was fraught with pain and depression. "Open-heart surgery hurts," he said. "But worse was the depression. I would find myself watching a comedy on TV and I would start to cry for no apparent reason. I would be writing a shopping list with my wife and I would start to cry. I would be reading the sports section of the paper and I would start to cry. And this went on for several months. The worst of all was when I was showering and I looked at all the scars on my legs where the veins were harvested. I would literally start to weep."

At the time I was watching this interview, one of my clients was about to undergo the same surgery. The

74 **John William Chancellor** (July 14, 1927–July 12, 1996) was a well-known American journalist, who spent most of his career associated with the NBC television network. His most famous career achievement was anchoring the *NBC Nightly News* from 1970 to 1982.

75 The **Johns Hopkins Hospital** is the teaching hospital and biomedical research facility of Johns Hopkins University School of Medicine, located in Baltimore, Maryland (USA).

76 **John William "Johnny" Carson** (October 23, 1925 – January 23, 2005) was an American television host and comedian, known as host of *The Tonight Show Starring Johnny Carson* for 30 years (1962–92).

coincidence of Chancellor and my client is what made me take such interest in the interview and to so clearly recall it for years afterward. I managed to forget the interview when it was my health at stake.

From my experience and from the experience of others I have figured out how to survive the depression. But first, here are some common warning signs:

Loss of appetite
Anxiety
Sense of hopelessness
Inability to concentrate
Inability to sleep
Lack of interest in almost everything
Inability to be with other people
Inability to be in crowds
Few things hold any interest
Reduced ability to experience pleasure
Pain, pain, pain
Worsening of pain
Headaches
Irrational behavior
Mood swings
Thoughts of suicide
Inability to recognize that you are depressed

Caregiver notes: There are many things you can be on the lookout for. Here is a list:

1. *Your patient does not laugh at things normally found funny.*
2. *Your patient does not eat what is usually a favorite dish.*
3. *When asked, "How are you?" your patient gives a lukewarm answer like, "OK."*

4. Your patient loses interest in outside activities.

5. When asked, "How are you?" your patient responds, "What do you mean by that?"

6. Etc.

Getting through the depression is a matter of survival and can reduce chances of a second heart attack by half!

Surviving Depression Strategies

Survival Strategy One: Solicit from those closest to you any sign of changing behavior. If you are exhibiting any of the above warning signs, there is a good chance you are already depressed.

Survival Strategy Two: Find a confidant to talk with. Spouses will usually be the ones that will demand you tell them everything before you talk with anyone else. Sometimes spouses are actually the worst confidants. There may be too much baggage in the long relationship for the spouse to be completely objective and responsive.

Caregiver notes: This is a hard thing to handle. You might have a strong feeling of anger right now given what your patient has put you through. The last thing you can afford to do is lay blame or take umbrage. You are going to have to grin and bear it.

Survival Strategy Three: Tell your doctor immediately if not sooner.

Caregiver notes: Remember you are the captain of the team. Your patient might not be able to recognize the symptoms, but you can. You need to tell the doctor if your patient does not. This might make your patient angry. Tough love is what is called for here.

Survival Strategy Four: Get twenty minutes of sun a day. Why is this so important? I must digress and tell you a short history lesson in American business.

In the 1880s, while U. S. Grant[77] was president, the US War Department (this was before it was renamed Department of Defense) undertook a study to determine the effect of diet on sailors and soldiers. The War Department selected a group of men where total control of what they ate and how much they ate could be exercised. The tests were conducted in three federal maximum-security prisons, the largest being Leavenworth. (At the conclusion of the tests, a general remarked, "We got our money's worth at Leavenworth.") The diseases under study were rickets, scurvy, and shingles, all of which could place whole units of soldiers out of commission and render them unable to fight.

The tests revealed that all the diseases could be prevented with daily small portions of protein, milk, if available, and citrus fruit. The test went on to say that a minimum daily exposure to the sun delivered the sunshine vitamins for free. It is nice to know that even then our War Department was watching the bucks.

Change of scene: John Patterson,[78] then the president and owner of National Cash Register,[79] read the report and immediately built the very first all glass factory in the world

---

77 **Ulysses S. Grant** (born **Hiram Ulysses Grant** (April 27, 1822 – July 23, 1885) was general-in-chief of the Union Army from 1864 to 1869 during the American Civil War and the 18th President of the United States from 1869 to 1877.

78 **John Henry Patterson** (December 13, 1844–May 7, 1922) was an industrialist and founder of the National Cash Register Company. He was a businessperson and salesperson.

79 **NCR Corporation** (NYSE: NCR) is a technology company specializing in products for the retail and financial sectors. Its main products are point-of-sale terminals, automated teller machines, check processing systems, barcode scanners, and business consumables. They also are one of the

in Dayton, Ohio, at the corner of K and Main streets. That factory was used continually for more than one hundred years. Patterson took this action because of a single paragraph in that report.[80]

The report stated that the twenty minutes a day of sun exposure not only made the prisoners healthier, it made them more malleable, more cooperative, and easier to control. So not only did Patterson build the factory, he made it mandatory that every morning at 10:00 a.m. all employees went to the east windows and stayed in the sun for twenty minutes. In the afternoon, the employees were sent to the west windows for another twenty minutes. This is where the twenty-minute morning and afternoon coffee breaks originated.

While Patterson lived, there were no employee problems that amounted to anything and the company was union free. Within two years of his death, on the other hand, a bean counter asked why such long breaks were given and no one remembered why the policy had been originated. The breaks were immediately reduced to ten minutes each and it was no longer necessary to go to the windows. A union was quickly elected in.

As it turns out, what the prisoner study demonstrated was the daily need for Vitamin D. The sunshine vitamin has extraordinary powers when it comes to combating depression and I'll have more to say on this subject in the discussion on the mental health issues associated with heart disease.

Survival Strategy Five: When you start to cry, really turn it on and allow yourself to feel. Do not try to stifle the crying jag or your emotions. Crying causes the body to release a group of hormones that will make you feel better when

largest providers of IT maintenance support services. From 1988 to 1997 they sponsored the NCR Book Award for nonfiction.

80 As told by S. C. Allyn in his autobiography, *My Fifty Years at NCR.*

the crying stops. It is your endocrine system that is causing the crying in response to your depression. Forget about the old nonsense that grown men don't cry. At this point in your recovery, crying is good for you, so really let it out. Watch a sad chick flick.

Caregiver notes: You can do this too.

Survival Strategy Six: If you don't have on, consider getting a pet. Many people find solace with a pet. Animals seem to have an extra sensory perception lacking in humans that allows the pet to recognize someone is feeling bad. When I came home from the hospital after each of the operations and I was at such a low point, it was the house cats that came to my rescue in some small way. All three of them jumped into the bed and nestled up to me. They had never done that before, never. And at night, when everyone's spirits sank, those cats would suddenly appear and jump onto the bed. It was like someone had said to the cats, "Go help that guy out," and they did.

In a recently released report, the experts concluded that having a pet helped people live longer happier lives. It turns out dogs are the best pets to lengthen life span. The principal reasons are dogs force people into a routine that requires exercise and dogs, more so than other animals, end up being considered one of the family. Of all those interviewed and tested, only 1 percent considered dogs as property.

Cats were next as the best pets. Cats don't enforce quite the same level of activity on their owners; however, cats provide a sense of tranquility and peace. It is also easier to hold a cat in your lap than it is to hold a medium-size dog. A purring cat is a reassuring presence. The only drawback with cats is their refusal to obey commands. I have seen many people walking dogs in my life; I have never seen anyone walking a cat.

Both pets give unconditional love. If you have one of each you receive the benefits of a dog, namely exercise (the twice daily walks) and blind obedience (a dog waits to wait and receive that little treat), and the benefit of cat, namely reassurance and tranquility. Nothing sleeps like a cat and nothing fetches like a dog. (Well, according to Jeff Foxworthy,[81] a well-trained husband fetches as well as a dog and it is not necessary to give a treat.)

Survival Strategy Seven: If you pray, pray. Many find solace in prayer. I have never been very big on this faith stuff but I cannot deny that while I was so sick I was told that many of my friends were praying for me. Just knowing there were people out there who cared enough about me to add me to their prayers made me feel better. As Frank Sinatra[82] said on numerous occasions, "Whatever gets you through the night."

This could just as well have been expressed as seeking some consolation in spiritual pursuits. According to psychoanalyst Carl Jung,[83] we are all connected by way of a "social unconsciousness." I don't really know what this means, but I do know that you get what you give. I don't even really know why I am including this. It just seems important to me.

Know this: A significant number of people with heart disease. Most open-heart surgery patients get depressed.

---

81 **Jeff Foxworthy** (born September 6, 1959) is an American stand-up comedian and actor.

82 **Francis Albert "Frank" Sinatra, Sr.** (December 12, 1915 – May 14, 1998), was an American singer and actor.

83 **Carl Gustav Jung** (26 July 1875 – 6 June 1961) was a Swiss psychiatrist, an influential thinker, and the founder of analytical psychology known as Jungian psychology.

You are going to be depressed. Recognize it, deal with it. Get help. Get over it.

Caregiver notes: You will not know what hits you when your patient gets depressed. Your patient will be non-responsive to almost everything. While raising a family, you got used to whiny kids. Whiny kids are a walk in the park compared to a heartsick, depressed patient. A depressed patient can't tell you what is wrong. It is not a case of the patient being uncooperative.

A depressed patient can't respond in a manner considered appropriate. You must report this to both the cardiologist and the primary care doctor. Be fore-warned. Depression retards the healing process. Worse, the docs might want to resort solely to the use of drugs to fight the depression. All of those drugs have serious side effects.

As it turns out, the American Heart Association has finally recognized the problem of depression in recovering from heart trauma. The AHA[84] has recently recommended that cardiologists start to look for depression in their patients by asking two questions:

1. In the past two weeks have you had little inter-est or pleasure in doing things?
2. Have you felt down, depressed, or hopeless?

Depression is three times more prevalent in heart trauma patients than the general population. The AHA went on to say that only about 50 percent of all cardiologists either look for or treat depression in their patients. Many patients, although diagnosed, are not treated. What is known is a depressed patient skips the medication, doesn't follow

---

84   Reported by the Associated Press, Jamie Stengle, reporter, and printed in the *Arizona Republic*, Tuesday, September 30, 2008.

the diet recommendations, doesn't exercise and doesn't partake in rehabilitation. The reporter, had more to say about this issue.

Fifty percent of cardiologists do not feel qualified to treat the severe depression. Nor do fifty percent recognize the problem. Many of the cardiologists refer the patient to a professional for treatment. The treatment can consist of drug therapy administered by your primary care doctor or a psychiatrist, or counseling from psychologists. Results are better when both therapies are used.

Psychiatrists are medical doctors and many do not do any counseling, other than to determine the extent of your illness. They are looking for a range of symptoms to establish a diagnosis. In my case the diagnosis was a current favorite of the day, bipolar behavior. Back in the day, this was called manic-depressive behavior. The symptom is great mood swings. You feel terrible or wonderful and nothing in between. Worse, the swings can occur in very short time spans.

Drugs are the treatment option of the psychiatrist. Once on the medications, they can be very hard to get off which was certainly my experience. There are those who might not agree with this observation. However, consider this: every drug used has a period of adjustment. Every drug, unless designed to be immediately effective, takes some period of time to start to demonstrate observable effect. Once you have adapted to the drug, it should not be immediately stopped. You may have to be weaned off the drug.

Talk, talk, talk is the treatment option of the psychologist. Once the talk begins, it can go on forever. More modern methods, such as cognitive behavioral therapy, can be very effective in a much shorter period of time. One way to help the psychologist help you is to have you and the caregiver know ahead of time what feelings and behaviors you'd like to change

(I find both psychiatry and psychology to be very strange. They both have no end date for their treatment. Every other medical specialty has deliverable results. Not the mental docs. In fact, it is in their best interest if you never get better. I'll have more to say about this subject in the section on anxiety. There are some caveats that can be offered. The deliverable result in psychiatry and psychology is the reduction or elimination of the symptoms of depression, anxiety, panic, etc. Research overwhelmingly shows that people do get better and terminate treatment successfully. If you are getting help, you might want to ask your professional what per cent of their patients actually stop seeing them.)

Those suffering untreated depression experience "poorer" outcomes. This is the euphemistic way of saying, "They die." The AHA made three primary recommendations on how to combat this ancillary killer to heart disease:

1. Diet
2. Take the medicine
3. Exercise

Where have I heard those three recommendations before?

Stephen R. Covey,[85] the author of *The 7 Habits of Highly Effective People*, writing an article for the Sunday weekly magazine *USA Weekend*,[86] reported on a study printed in the medical journal *Nature Reviews Neuroscience* about the effect and affect of Vitamin D. Here is what Covey, the advice guru, wrote:

"A low level of vitamin D—the 'sunshine vitamin'—can put a damper on your mood. Depressed people had 14 percent less vitamin D in their blood than non-depressed

---

85 **Stephen R. Covey** (born October 24, 1932).

86 *USA Weekend* as a supplement to the *Arizona Republic*, January 2–4, 2009

people in a Dutch study of 1,282 seniors. So load up on D: while you're improving your mood, you'll be helping your bones too. Adequate levels of vitamin D also are vital for calcium absorption and bone health.

"But don't stop there. You can eat your way to a happier day. Omega-3 fatty acids found in foods such as salmon, walnuts, flaxseed, scallops, and cod-liver oil also help fight depression, mood disorders, schizophrenia, and dementia."

Stress goes hand in hand with the depression. The stress causes a rise in your blood pressure. The rise in the blood pressure makes you feel more anxious and the increased anxiety makes you more depressed; the spiral just keeps going on and on. There are many ways to deal with this. The first is to get a pill to combat the tension. This is the path of least resistance and requires you to do nothing other than to shell out the bucks and remember to take the pills. As it turns out, taking a pill is the least desirable way to cope with the problem. We will spend some amount of time on this subject.

Once again, late in the cycle of writing this, I got to learn something new about stress—just when I thought I knew it all. Once again, it was *Nova* that showed me what an ignorant so-and-so I am. That program, about the effect of stress, studied three separate groups: a group of bureaucrats in London, a troop of baboons in Africa, and a large group of macaque monkeys in a zoo. I find it so reassuring that we can so successfully be compared to bureaucrats, baboons, and monkeys, don't you?

The primates were chosen thanks in large measure to their similarities to humans. We share similar biology, genetics, and social systems. No, the program did not say we descended from the baboons and monkeys. It did say we are genetic cousins with very common biology and physiology. As the study demonstrated, we also share very similar social pressures and stress. I found the program both enlightening and disconcerting.

The program focused on a study about the social pressures. All three groups had the same kinds of social pressures. Here is the list:

- The role of dominant or type A individuals in doling out stress. It appears the type A rulers enjoyed passing out the lumps.
- The role of the subordinate types in receiving the grief. It appears the subordinate members had to accept the bad behavior or be either physically abused, murdered, or banished.
- The behavior of the type A's toward females, which was one of continual harassment and physical beatings.
- The requirement of the groups to groom and give pleasure to the dominant males.

In the London study, one bureaucrat was so abused by his boss he had a mental breakdown. The man was out of work for six months trying to get his life back together. When he finally did return, he found he had a new supervisor. Without going into all the details of how his new supervisor treated him, the treatment was so superior in all aspects, the bureaucrat's performance improved. This proved something we have all always known—good bosses get good performance from their employees.

The baboon study covered a tragedy that occurred to one of the targeted troops. Ten years into the study one troop took to feasting on the garbage of a tourist hotel. The dining was limited to the dominant males. They all got TB and died. Fortunately, for the rest of the troop, the hotel cleaned up its act and stopped leaving garbage for the baboons to eat. The scientists studying the troop believed the troop would quickly disband or be killed off by other baboons. That is not what happened.

The remaining males were, as the scientists said in technical terms, "nice guys." They did not abuse the females, nor did they get yucks in passing out lumps. Instead, they were kind to the ladies and spent the day passing out pleasure (this is called grooming in baboon terms) and receiving pleasure in kind. This behavior has persisted for another twenty years.

In baboon society, it is customary for young adult baboons to leave one troop and go become part of another troop. When a new baboon comes into the "good guy" troop, he gets a rude awakening as to what is tolerated behavior. If the new baboons exhibit that bad old type A behavior, they are shunned and no one gives them any pleasure. In less than six months, they get the idea and modify their behavior to fit in.

The group of macaque monkeys exhibited very similar behavior as the baboons. Having the monkeys confined to a large enclosure provided the ability to make some other very interesting observations. It made it easy to see the difference in body shape and size of the different monkeys. Just like in human society, some of the monkeys were fat and some thin. You know the expression fat, dumb, and happy? Well the study showed that fat and happy did not go together.

In fact, fat and unhappy was the observable characteristic. The most abused monkeys were the fattest monkeys. Those monkeys were compulsive eaters, constantly on the alert for superior members of the group, and literally jumping at the least disturbance. The thinnest monkeys were those that received the most grooming and most favorable attention from the rest of the group.

Brain scans revealed the truth in all three studies. There is a "pleasure" center in the brain of all higher primates. In all cases, those receiving the most pleasure had high stimulus in that section of the brain. Humans, baboons, and monkeys all had the same result. Those receiving lots of pleasure had high stimulus. Those receiving little pleasure had low stimulus. High stress equaled no pleasure equaled no stimulus.

The studies examined the changes in body shape caused by the social pressures, and the enzymes the body produced in response to the stress. The major conclusion of all the studies is this: stress is a really bad thing. I wonder how much money was spent to get to that conclusion. I'll bet you couldn't figure that out for yourself. Well, so much for the cheap shot. Here are the important findings:

- Stress causes the body to produce an undesirable enzyme that forces the body to store fat around the middle. This is the worst possible place to store fat. This is the worst possible fat to store. This is the fat that causes big insulin spikes.
- Stress prevents happiness.
- Stress promotes unreasonable fear. (I don't know about this. It would seem to me that if you are in constant danger of being beat up on both physically and mentally than maybe the fear is not unreasonable.)
- There is no such thing as "good" stress when it is being induced by duress. (There are many who will say there is "good" stress. This is related to stress related to adrenalin surge in reaction to the need to perform. The study did not concern itself with this type of stress.)
- Stressed individuals lead shorter, unhappier lives than those handing out the stress.

One way to fight stress is to get as much pleasure as you can from as many sources as you can; that pleasure should not be at someone else's expense. Another way is to get off your backside and get moving. The exercise will combat the stress. The exercise will release the endorphins, making you feel physically better and emotionally lighter.

The euphoric feeling will relieve the stress; bring your blood pressure down, and save you the money for the drugs.

Caregiver notes: You will be as stressed as the patient, if not more so. Not only do you have to cope with the patient's mental illness, you must look out for yourself. It is hard, unrewarding work caring for a heart patient. Too often, the patient is in no position to appreciate what is being done. Accept this fact. Your patient would say thank you if he were able to understand what was going on. The patient is not capable of care recognition at this point.

The patient's behavior can be very wearing on you. You must look out for yourself during this time. You must not accept the patient's bad behavior as being your fault.

I have saved one of the worst symptoms for the end: Anxiety. This is not a Mel Brooks[87] send-up of Alfred Hitchcock[88] movies. This is a real terror and one that is extremely hard to combat. The easiest path of resistance is to once again take a pill. The medicine used to combat the anxiety, and simultaneously attack the stress and the depression is called a psychotropic. Once you start taking these drugs, effective as they may be, you need to be on guard for dependency.

From experience, I can explain a sequence or events once these behavior-altering meds are used. I became convinced I was crazy. I was also taking prednisone, an anabolic steroid, to combat the pleural inflammations I described above. If you are advised to take these medications, I would advise getting a second opinion.

---

87 **Melvin "Mel" Kaminsky** (born June 28, 1926). Better known by his stage name Mel Brooks, is an American film director, screenwriter, composer, lyricist, comedian, actor, and producer, best known as a creator of broad film farces and comic parodies.

88 **Sir Alfred Joseph Hitchcock**, KBE (13 August 1899 – 29 April 1980) was a British filmmaker and producer who pioneered many techniques in the suspense and psychological thriller genres.

An extremely undesirable side effect of steroids is RAGE. Steroids totally screw up your endocrine system. I am not a physically big man. Yet, while taking those drugs, I found myself willing to fight much bigger and much younger men. I turned on one very large young man in a retail store. He must have seen the insanity in my eyes and quickly backed down. If he had opted to fight, he would have killed me. I was asked to leave the premises. The only reason I did leave was I had to find a restroom—diuretics.

However, that was not the end of the story. I got progressively worse. I was taking the steroid and to combat the side effect of that, I was taking two tranquilizers and a strong sleeping drug. I began to entertain serious thoughts of suicide. Every drug I was prescribed had a side effect that required another drug to counteract it. I was taking twenty or so medications a day. I needed a program to keep track of what drug I should take when. What a mess.

Then in August of 2003, I'd had enough. My wife went out to shop and I went and took handfuls of the tranquilizers and sleeping meds. As Hamlet[89] said, "Perchance to dream." At that point, I only wanted out. I woke up in the hospital. My pacemaker kept me alive. My wife found me passed out on the bed when she came home and called 911. I was restrained. I was mad I was still alive.

It took me more than a year to get my feet back under me. I was diagnosed as bipolar with the appropriate medicine cocktail to help me maintain. Then one day I'd had enough of that. I looked around at the group in my therapy session and realized what was going on with all of them and with me. It was that day that I started to heal myself.

My psychologist said something very interesting to me. He said I needed to recognize there was no scientific evidence that what others were seeing in me was false.

---

89 **The Tragedy of Hamlet, Prince of Denmark**, or more simply **Hamlet**, is a tragedy by William Shakespeare, believed to have been written between 1599 and 1601.

Translation: what others were seeing is what I was. The problems were mine, not theirs. Oh, damn.

In looking at other seriously depressed people, whom I was seeing a lot of in those days, I realized they were not getting over whatever it was that made them depressed. I had lost a lot of ego when I got sick. I had to get over me. I saw it all in a blinding flash. I went to my internist and made him go through the list of meds, one by one, and explain why I was taking them. That very day, in my internist's office, I stopped taking all but those few drugs I absolutely had to take for the health of my heart. I quit every other drug.

The psychiatrist did not like this. He said I would end up in the hospital again. I didn't. I never saw him again.

When I explained how what the psychologist had said had made me see the light, he thought I was on the right track and bid me a fond farewell.

It took about six weeks for all the drugs to finally exit my system.

You probably remember the big stink Tom (*Top Gun*) Cruise[90] made about how depression did not require doctors or medications to be cured. It is just not so. Depression is a very real danger, and when united with anxiety and stress, you are hitting the trifecta. However, having said that, there are some things you can do to help cure yourself.

The first two things you can do are (1) stop drinking sugared, caffeinated beverages; (2) get your vitamin D as above; and (3) once again, get off your butt. Coffee has become a national obsession. I don't drink the stuff myself because I never really liked it. But I did drink Coca-Cola, the all American soda pop. Beverages that have both sugar, whether added as an ingredient while being concocted,

---

90 **Thomas Cruise Mapother IV** (born July 3, 1962), better known by his screen name of **Tom Cruise**, is an American actor and film producer.

or added at the table prior to drinking, and caffeine, ramp up your body.

The sugar gives you an immediate lift followed by a sugar low and the caffeine tells the endocrine system to get busy for work, only you are not going to do any work. The two ingredients together ramp up your body for nothing and that makes you anxious. Mix that freshly created anxiety with the already existing stress and depression and, boy howdy…give that person another ride on the roller coaster of terror.

Now let us add the fear of the unknown into the equation. You are going to be afraid before, during, and after any serious coronary procedure. It is part of the job description. It is right there on page nine of the handbook for chronic heart disease patients. You didn't get one? Ask your doc for one. A word of warning, the doc will probably look at you as if you have just grown a second head. Or he may tell you about this book.

Perseverance Dictums

Well, Hoss, let's round 'em up and put 'em away. Getting better and staying well is a matter of perseverance. Here are some dictums that work for me and should work for you. I am nobody special. All I have going for me is my experience and my willingness to persevere. Did I ever mention what caused me to learn all of the above, other than how I went through that first heart attack? I was only fifty-eight at that time. Everything was taken away from me in virtually a single event. So you can take it to the bank that I have lived through everything I speak about here.

Dictum One: Live the diet.

Dictum Two: Exercise.

Dictum Three: Get educated about your drugs and follow the protocols.

Dictum Four: Don't watch any daytime TV. That crap will fry your brains.

Dictum Five: Go to library and read two or three books a week.

Dictum Six: Exercise your brain. Do word and number puzzles.

Dictum Seven: Laugh and laugh hard. Laugh until your sides hurt and you can't catch your breath.

Dictum Eight: Sing, even if you can't carry a tune in a bucket or, as Momma Cass[91] sang, "Even if no one else sings along."

Dictum Nine: Give and get pleasure. The more pleasure you can give, the more you are likely to get. If bureaucrats, baboons, and monkeys can do it, so can you. (I wonder if Cole Porter[92] could have written a song like that.)

Dictum Ten: You should eat a piece or two of dark chocolate (not milk chocolate) a couple of times a week. The only admonition for this is if you have diabetes.

Dictum Eleven: Live long, live well, and prosper—Peace. (True story: My wife and I met Leonard Nimoy[93] [you know,

---

91 **Cass Elliot** (September 19, 1941 – July 29, 1974), born **Ellen Naomi Cohen**, was a noted American singer, best remembered as **Mama Cass** of the pop quartet The Mamas & the Papas.

92 **Cole Albert Porter** (June 9, 1891 – October 15, 1964) was an American composer and songwriter from Peru, Indiana.

93 **Leonard Simon Nimoy** (born March 26, 1931) is an American actor, film director, poet, musician, and photographer. He played the character

Spock of *Star Trek* fame] in, of all places, outside the See's Candy Store [show me somebody who doesn't like See's Candy and I will show you someone who is un-American] at the Arrowhead Mall. He had just bought some See's Candy to take home with him. As I say above in Dictum Ten, eat some dark chocolate; it's good for you. I believe anything good enough for Spock is good enough for me.)

Your life is now one of give-and-take. If you don't want to exercise, OK, don't eat that day. If you want the extra salt, OK, don't have any for the next several days. If you want that extra LDL fat in your diet one day, OK, don't have any LDL fats for the next several days. If you don't feel like taking the drugs you are supposed to take, when you are supposed to take them, OK, don't and see what happens and suffer the consequences.

You are solely responsible for your care and well-being. Not your loved ones. Not your friends. Not your spouse. Especially not your doctor. And certainly not me. You and you alone have to carry the burden. So, as I wrote early on, if you are not going to accept full responsibility and follow all the rules, then don't follow any of them. That way you will die sooner and others will have more time to get the care they deserve because they follow the rules.

The decision is yours.

Caregiver notes: My patient really does follow all the rules. He cheats but he follows the rules of cheating. At one time, he thought in terms of living, maybe for another year, at best. Not anymore. He knows if he follows the rules and takes responsibility for his actions, his life span is as undetermined as anyone else's. He can still be a pain in the butt, but then so can everyone else.

---

of Spock on *Star Trek*, an American television series that ran for three seasons from 1966 to 1969, and he reprised the role in the movie sequels (most recently 2009's *Star Trek*) and the follow-up series *Star Trek: The Next Generation*.

Lastly, now that he is doing so well, he does thank me for living with and putting up with it all.

Postscript

It seems to me that no matter how good your work, somebody can do better. I no sooner come up with what I have learned on how to live with CHF when *Men's Health Magazine* comes up with ten ways to live forever. As Mel Allen[94] would have said, "How about that, sports fans?"

How to live forever is a lot longer than I would claim. As for me, I'll take a pass on forever and settle for getting by on a daily basis. Herewith is their list. You might quickly notice there is not a single mention of exercise. My guess is *Men's Health Magazine* suggests you live like a mushroom. You know, in the dark and covered with fertilizer. I have added a few thoughts.

Top 10 Ways to Live Forever

No drugs. No bypasses. No scars. Just solid DIY advice on how to keep your heart pumping.

1. By the Editors of *Men's Health*. **Grill a steak.** You may think it's bad for your heart, but you'd be wrong. Beef contains immunity-boosting selenium as well as homocysteine-lowering B vitamins. And up to 50 percent of the fat is the heart-healthy monounsaturated variety.

---

94 **Mel Allen** (February 14, 1913 – June 16, 1996) was an American sportscaster, best known for his long tenure as the primary play-by-play announcer for the New York Yankees. During the peak of his career in the 1940s, 1950s, and 1960s, Allen was arguably the most prominent member of his profession, his voice familiar to millions, and will forever be known as the one and only "Legendary Voice of the New York Yankees." In his later years, he gained a second professional life as the first host of *This Week in Baseball*.

I have pondered this. The recommended amount of red meat allowable on the heart-healthy diets is approximately three ounces a month, a portion the size of a deck of cards. As to the selenium, you can get that equivalent in a good multipurpose vitamin. I have discovered buffalo. Buffalo has one quarter the LDL fat of beef and all the good stuff. If you can find it, try it.

2. **Tell your wife to butt out.** People who are exposed to cigarette smoke for just 30 minutes, three times a week, have a 26 percent greater risk of developing heart disease than people who rarely encounter secondhand smoke.

If you are worried about heart disease and either of you smokes, then you already know what I think about that—MORON.

3. **Take aspirin.** Regular aspirin consumption cuts the risk of CAD by 28 percent in people who have never had a heart attack or stroke.

Good advice; however, it is not a good idea to take aspirin based on the advice of a magazine. I take 81 milligrams of aspirin a day to help thin my blood, but then I also take Coumadin. Aspirin can also eat away at the stomach lining if used on a regular basis. It is best to check with your doc.

4. **Drink more tea.** Men who drink two cups of tea a day are 25 percent less likely to die of heart disease than guys who rarely touch the stuff. The reason: flavonoids in the tea, which not only improve blood vessels' ability to relax, but also thin the blood, reducing clotting.

Yep, I guess tea is a good thing. However, tea contains a significant amount of caffeine. If you are a regular hi-test coffee drinker, this might not be such a good idea. If you are going to take this advice, I suggest you drink decaffeinated tea.

5. **Touch her.** Ten minutes of skin-to-skin contact (hand-holding, hugs) with your mate can help keep your blood pressure and pulse from spiking during stressful times, according to University of North Carolina researchers.
You betcha, Kemo Sabe.

6. **Go fishing for tuna.** Omega-3 fats in tuna help strengthen heart muscle, lower blood pressure, and prevent clotting—as well as reduce levels of potentially deadly inflammation in the body.

This falls in the category of almost right. Fish, other than fried, in general, is a good idea. There are four fishes that are better for you than tuna and they are mackerel, herring, sardines, and salmon. These four fairly bristle with high omega-3 oil that is good for your heart. They are also considered "rough" fish. Freshwater fish don't pack the power of that oil.

7. **Pair up.** Married men are less likely to die of heart disease than bachelors. Scientists looked at men with mildly high blood pressure and found that after three years of marriage, the happily married men had healthier hearts than their unmarried brothers.

"So why would this be true?" you may ask. How many single men do you know that can cook? Single men eat fast food much more often than married men with wives that cook. I have no statistics to back this up. Only observation. Of course, companionship and love "ain't" bad things either.

8. **Adopt a dog.** All that love ("You're a good boy, yes you are!") and aggravation ("Bad dog! Don't eat Daddy's crab dip!") makes your heart more adaptable and better able to deal with the stress that can lead to heart disease.

I am amazed at how they get it almost right. The real benefit of a dog is the exercise the dog's regime forces on you. Walking the pooch twice or more a day forces you to get off your butt and out of the house. That motion is not only a stress reliever, it gets the blood pumping. The dog appreciates it as well and rewards you with affection.

9. **Rinse, brush.** Rinse your mouth with mouthwash and toothpaste that has antibacterial properties. They'll reduce oral bacteria, which can decrease your risk of a heart attack by 200–300 percent.

Hard to argue with that, although I have no idea where they get their statistics. The point of the matter is there is a direct line between your teeth and your heart and anything you can do to reduce the amount of infection in your mouth is a step toward a heart-healthy lifestyle.

10. Make friends at work. Men with the most work friends also have the lowest heart rates and healthiest blood-pressure levels, even during times of stress.

I don't know about friends from work. My experience with friends from work is not so good. It seemed to me that when we were together we spent a lot of time speaking about work. The last thing I wanted to talk about away from work was work. The real issue is the value of friends with whom you share like experiences, backgrounds, cultures, or interests. My observation seems to lead to the conclusion that real friends, the ones you can count on in times of crisis, are few and far between. Also, friends from work come and go and can be as changeable as the seasons. Worse, those friendships seem to crumble into dust if you get promoted over your friends, or vice versa.

Now you can go back and reread the thirteen signs you will live a long time. Peace and "How 'bout them Cubs?"[95]

---

95 I just can't imagine anyone not knowing about the Chicago Cubs. The Chicago Cubs and the Brooklyn Dodgers, when the Dodgers were still "The Bums," are probably responsible for more depression, grief, and heart attacks than any other cause known to humanity. Of course that is just my opinion. You won't find this in any medical journal. Just ask any fan.

Extra Short Complete Summary

Here are all sixty thousand or so words of the book condensed into about seven hundred and forty-three words:

Measurement Mandates

Mandate 1: The inventors of the tests determine the measurements.

Mandate 2: All units of measurement are arbitrarily assigned.

Mandate 3: Measurement meaning is based on population testing results.

Mandate 4: Results of the measurement metrics are indicators of patient state of health.

Mandate 5: Medical metrics are universally understood.

Mandate 6: No single measurement determines the state of the patient's health.

Mandate 7: The greater the number of tests, the more certain is the accuracy of the diagnosis.

Mandate 8: The greater the number of tests, the greater the costs to be borne by the health care system and the patient.

Mandate 9: You get what you pay for.

Testing Truths

Truth One: Testing is mandatory and may be neither overlooked nor not done.

Truth Two: Not performing tests can lead to misdiagnosis or death.

Truth Three: With no testing, there is no measurement.

Truth Four: With no measurement there is no comparison, and with no comparison there is no conclusion.

Truth Five: Testing delivers the baseline metrics that constitute the answers to the interrogatives.

Truth Six: You can't learn about what you do not test for.

Truth Seven: The most important test is probably the one that was overlooked.

Caregiver Basics

1. *Stay optimistic*
2. *Get educated*
3. *Have patience with the patient*
4. *Keep everything extra clean*
5. *Make tender loving care your stock in trade*
6. *Get help*
7. *Change your life philosophies and expectations*
8. *Get prepared*
9. *Stay the course*
10. *Exercise appropriate discipline*

Philosophical Tenets

Tenet One: Acknowledge the situation for what it really is.

Tenet Two: Accept ownership.

Tenet Three: Agree on what has to be done to move on.

Tenet Four: Commit to making the changes.

Tenet Five: Change your life.

Tenet Six: Prepare for the future.

Rules of Acceptance

First rule of acceptance: It's your fault.

Second rule of acceptance: You are too damn fat.

Third rule of acceptance: If you smoke, you are a moron.

Fourth rule of acceptance: The changes you must make are for the rest of your life.

Fifth rule of acceptance: You are not alone.

Sixth rule of acceptance: You need someone to talk to about what you are going through.

Seventh rule of acceptance: Follow all the directions your health care professionals give you.

Eighth rule of acceptance: Take it all personally.

Ninth rule of acceptance: Get educated.

Tenth rule of acceptance: You are going to need a support network to help you heal.

Eleventh rule of acceptance: The path to recovery is almost identical to the path traveled by someone coping with the loss of a loved one.

Science Laws

First Law of Science: NO SALT!

Second Law of Science: NO FAT!

Third Law of Science: LEARN ABOUT SUBSTITUTION.

Fourth Law of Science: GET EDUCATED.

Fifth Law of Science: EASTABLISH AND STICK TO YOUR DIET.

Prescription Proscriptions

Proscription One: Know what you are taking and why.

Proscription Two: Take the medications as prescribed.

Proscription Three: All drugs are toxic and may have side effects.

Proscription Four: Drugs are not "bulletproof" vests.

Proscription Five: If something changes, immediately tell your doctor.

Proscription Six: Make sure you renew your prescriptions in plenty of time.

Proscription Seven: Do not start arbitrarily taking any over-the-counter medications.

Proscription Eight: Carry a list of all your drugs, dosages, and directions at all times when you are out and about.

Rules of Participation

First Rule of Participation: Exercise is not easy.

Second Rule of Participation: You must take small steps at the outset and you must find the exercise that suits your temperament.

Third Rule of Participation: The best exercises for old broken-down heart patients like us are **LOW-IMPACT** exercises.

Fourth Rule of Participation: Arrange a daily exercise schedule with a start and finish time.

Fifth Rule of Participation: Combine low-impact aerobic exercise with light weight exercises.

Sixth Rule of Participation: Set your routine and stick with it.

Seventh Rule of Participation: Always start and end your routine with a standard set of stretching exercises.

Surviving Depression Strategies

Survival Strategy One: Solicit from those closest to you any sign of changing behavior.

Survival Strategy Two: Find a confidant to talk with.

Survival Strategy Three: Tell your doctor immediately if not sooner.

Survival Strategy Four: Get twenty minutes of sun a day.

Survival Strategy Five: When you start to cry, really turn it on.

Survival Strategy Six: Get a pet.

Survival Strategy Seven: If you pray, pray.

Perseverance Dictums

Dictum One: Live the diet.

Dictum Two: Exercise.

Dictum Three: Get educated about your drugs and follow the protocols.

Dictum Four: Don't watch any daytime TV.

Dictum Five: Go to the library and read two or three books a week.

Dictum Six: Exercise your brain. Do word and number puzzles.

Dictum Seven: Laugh and laugh hard. Laugh until your sides hurt and you can't catch your breath.

Dictum Eight: Sing, even if you can't carry a tune.

Dictum Nine: Give and get pleasure.

Dictum Ten: You should eat a piece or two of dark chocolate (not milk chocolate) a couple of times a week.

Dictum Eleven: Live long, live well, and prosper—Peace.

Epilogue

Last Fable

A person goes to a doctor and complains about being short of breath and suffering occasional chest pains. The patient says to the doctor, "To be honest, it is hard for me to move my ass." The doctor examines the person including the traditional weight and blood pressure measurements. The doctor then says to the patient, stop smoking, lose twenty-five pounds, exercise an hour a day, and come back to see me in ninety days.

The patient complies and stops smoking, exercises, and loses twenty-five pounds. The patient returns in ninety days and tells the doctor he's feeling a little better. The doctor, after examining and measuring and testing the patient, says, "You are making good progress. Take this medicine, continue not to smoke and continue to exercise and lose fifteen pounds and don't eat foods high in cholesterol and salt. Eat more fish. See me in ninety days."

The patient complies. The patient returns in ninety days. The patient is feeling very good. The patient's energy levels have gone way up. The color has returned to the patient's cheeks. The patient says to the doctor, "I feel so much better. You are a miracle worker." The doctor says, "Continue to not smoke, continue to exercise, lose ten more pounds, continue to eat more fish, and don't eat high cholesterol and salty foods. Come back in six months." The patient says, "Verily you are a god."

Moral: Doctors help those that help themselves.

~

...And the heartbeat goes on...

Have you ever finished reading a book or watching a movie and thought to yourself, "What happens next?" We thought when we finished writing the book that would be the end of the story. As it is evolving, it appears that finishing the writing is only the beginning. You must understand this is coming from a guy who is extremely lazy and whose idea of work is, well, come to think of it, I have no idea of work. I had laid down my tools and I am off the clock forever. Fat chance.

We have had to open a Web site. In fact, we had to take several names and you can find us by using Google or any other browser for that matter and entering simplehand. Or just go to www.simplehand.org. The purpose of our site is to provide a source for almost anything you want to know about living with heart disease or the other chronic diseases we wrote about in this book.

On the Web site you will be able to read our vision statement and mission statement. That will pretty much explain what we are about. The principal thrust of the site will be to give ongoing information about nutrition and diet, exercise, care giving, and, of course, heart disease and other chronic diseases. I wouldn't be surprised if a cartoon doesn't sneak in there somewhere.

In addition, we will be starting a blog, one that we hope will be different from the others. The site will explain how to become part of the discussion.

Of course, it does not stop there. Twitter is necessary. Facebook, U Tube, and Linkedin all play a part in the ever-expanding world of information dissemination. Who knows where it will end. I can tell you this: if it is not easy, I am not doing it.

Even doctors like this book. Their reasoning is simple. The book says everything they would like to say. The groundswell is starting toward managing for better outcomes and some early adopters are using the book as part of their outreach programs for cardiac patients. You might ask if your health care providers even have an outreach program.

Anyway, it is the way of the world. Education and information is all. Please join us.

Oh, and thank you very much for buying and reading this book.

☙

Glossary

A

Anesthesiologist – a physician who specializes in anesthesiology.

Anesthesia machine – The anaesthetic machine (or anesthesia machine in America) is used by anesthesiologists to support the administration of anaesthesia. The most common type of anaesthetic machine in use in the developed world is the continuous-flow anaesthetic machine, which is designed to provide an accurate and continuous supply of medical gases (such as oxygen and nitrous oxide), mixed with an accurate concentration of anaesthetic vapour (such as isoflurane), and deliver this to the patient at a safe pressure and flow. Modern machines incorporate a ventilator, suction unit, and patient-monitoring devices. Source - Wickipedia

Angiogram – an x-ray produced by angiography

Angiograph – x-ray examination of blood vessels or lymphatics following injection of a radiopaque substance.

Anti-cholesterol – is a naturally occurring antibody to cholesterol produced by mammals. It is believed that this antibody serves a 'housekeeping' or protective role for the host animal, helping to protect the animal from harmful forms of cholesterol such as LDL and VLDL.

Modes of Action

An immunoglobulin protein, *anti-cholesterol* may be found both in circulation as well as in the digestive tract.

- In circulation, this antibody binds selectively to the small, dense, oxidized cholesterol-rich LDL particles that are known to contribute to the development of atherosclerosis. The antibody does not bind the good forms of cholesterol such as HDL.
- In the gastrointestinal tract, the antibody acts as a cholesterol absorption inhibitor. The antibody selectively binds to cholesterol-rich micelles and prevents their uptake by the intestinal enterocyte. The antibody-bound micelle is then removed through fecal clearance.

Arrhythmia – any disturbance in the rhythm of the heartbeat.

Atherosclerosis – a common form of arteriosclerosis in which fatty substances form a deposit of plaque on the inner lining of arterial walls.

Atrial fibrillation – *noun* very rapid uncoordinated contractions of the atria of the heart resulting in a lack of synchronism between heartbeat and pulse beat called also *auricular fibrillation*

B

Blood pressure – The pressure of the blood against the inner walls of the blood vessels, varying in different parts of the body during different phases of contraction of the heart and under different conditions of health, exertion, etc. *Abbreviation:* BP

Bypass – is a type of heart surgery. It's sometimes called CABG (cabbage). The surgery reroutes, or bypasses, blood around clogged arteries to improve the supply of blood and oxygen to the heart. ... Cardiopulmonary bypass with a pump oxygenator (heart-lung machine) is used for most coronary bypass graft operations

C

Cardiac care unit – Immediately after having a major heart surgery, it's typical for patients to be moved into the cardiac care unit, or CCU. Find out what this means for you and your family. ... The equivalent of an intensive care unit, or ICU, which is for critically ill patients with other types ... Many different cardiac medications may be given. This may also be called a Cardiac Intensive Care Unit. In some hospitals, the cardiac care unit is a step down in care after the patient has gotten through the initial period immediately following surgery.

Cardiac disease – See heart disease below.

Cardiac surgeon – A cardiac surgeon is a surgeon who performs cardiac surgery—operative procedures on the heart and great vessels.

Cardiologist – the study of the heart and its functions in health and disease.

Caregiver – a person who cares for someone who is sick or disabled or an adult who cares for an infant or child.

Cholesterol – A white crystalline substance, $C_{27}H_{45}OH$, found in animal tissues and various foods, that is normally synthesized by the liver and is important as a constituent of cell membranes and a precursor to steroid hormones. Its level in the bloodstream can influence the pathogenesis of certain conditions, such as the development of atherosclerotic plaque and coronary artery disease

CHF – Heart failure (also known as congestive heart failure) is a condition in which the heart is not able to pump enough blood. Medication may help, but surgery may be needed, including heart transplant surgery. Devices such as an intra-aortic balloon pump or ventricular assist device may help until a donor heart becomes available.

CICU – See CCU

Clinical pharmacist – Clinical pharmacy is the branch of Pharmacy where pharmacists provide patient care that optimizes the use of medication and promotes health, wellness and disease prevention. Clinical pharmacists care for patients in all health care settings but the clinical pharmacy movement initially began inside hospitals and clinics. Clinical pharmacists often collaborate with physicians and other healthcare professionals.

Congestive heart failure – See CHF

Chronic Obstructive Pulmonary Disease – (COPD Any of various lung diseases leading to poor pulmonary aeration, including emphysema and chronic bronchitis.

Coronary artery disease – A condition (as sclerosis or thrombosis) that reduces the blood flow through the coronary arteries to the heart muscle called also *coronary disease, coronary heart disease*

Coumadin – a brand name for warfarin. See Warfarin

D

Diabetes – Any of several disorders characterized by increased urine production. Usually typified by increased urine production caused by inadequate secretion of vasopressin by the pituitary gland. This is a disorder of carbohydrate metabolism, usually occurring in genetically predisposed individuals, characterized by inadequate production or utilization of insulin and resulting in excessive amounts of glucose in the blood and urine, excessive thirst, weight loss, and in some cases progressive destruction of small blood vessels leading to such complications as infections and gangrene of the limbs or blindness.

Also called **Type I diabetes, insulin-dependent diabetes**, *juvenile diabetes*, a severe form of diabetes mellitus in which insulin production by the beta cells of the pancreas is impaired, usually resulting in dependence on externally administered insulin, the onset of the disease typically occurring before the age of 25.

Also called **Type II diabetes, non-insulin-dependent diabetes, *adult-onset diabetes*,** maturity onset diabetes, a mild, sometimes asymptomatic form of diabetes mellitus characterized by diminished tissue sensitivity to insulin and sometimes by impaired beta cell function, exacerbated by obesity and often treatable by diet and exercise.

Diuretic – increasing the volume of the urine excreted, as by a medicinal substance.

E

Echocardiogram – In each case, an ultrasound **machine** is used. With the help of a microphone-shaped device (known as a transducer) ultrasound waves are created and beamed through water. ... An echocardiogram can be obtained in a physician's office or in the hospital. For a resting echocardiogram (in contrast to a stress **echo** or TEE, EKG/blood pressure monitors

Echocardiograph – The probe of an echocardiography machine contains a transducer, which emits and records ultrasound. ... By measuring the time it takes for the return echo to reach the probe and comparing it against a calibrated time, one can measure the distance between the probe and the interface. The result is a one-dimensional display.

Edema – An effusion of serous fluid into the interstices of cells in tissue spaces or into body cavities.

F

FDA – Food and Drug 'Administration

Heart attack – *damage* to an area of heart muscle that is deprived of oxygen, usually due to blockage of a diseased coronary artery, typically accompanied by chest pain radiating down one or both arms, the severity of the attack varying with the extent and location of the damage; myocardial heart disease Heart disease or cardiopathy is an umbrella term for a variety for different diseases affecting the heart. As of 2007, it is the leading cause of death in the United States, England, Canada and Wales, killing one person every 34 seconds in the United States alone.

heart failure

1. A condition in which the heart fatally ceases to function.
2. Also called **congestive heart failure.** a condition in which the heart fails to pump adequate amounts of blood to the tissues, resulting in accumulation of blood returning to the heart from the veins, and often accompanied by distension of the ventricles, edema, and shortness of breath.

Heart-lung machine – a device through which blood is shunted temporarily for oxygenation during surgery, while the heart or a lung is being repaired.

High blood pressure – elevation of the arterial blood pressure or a condition resulting from it; hypertension.

Hypertension – See high blood pressure.

Hyperlipidemia – excessive amounts of fat and fatty substances in the blood; lipemia

I

INR – International Normalized Ratio

Internist (primary caregivers) – a physician specializing in the diagnosis and non-surgical treatment of diseases

Intravenous lines – Intravenous therapy or IV therapy is the giving of liquid substances directly into a vein. It can be intermittent or continuous; continuous administration is called an intravenous drip. The word intravenous simply means "within a vein", but is most commonly used to refer to IV therapy.

L

Lipids – any of a group of organic compounds that are greasy to the touch, insoluble in water, and soluble in alcohol and ether: lipids comprise the fats and other esters with analogous properties and constitute, with proteins and carbohydrates, the chief structural components of living cells.

O

Open-heart surgery – surgery performed on the exposed heart while a heart-lung machine pumps and oxygenates the blood and diverts it from the heart.

Operating theater – a room in a hospital equipped for the performance of surgical operations; "great care is taken to keep the operating rooms aseptic"

M

Mitochondria – A structure in the cytoplasm of all cells except bacteria in which food molecules (sugars, fatty acids, and amino acids) are broken down in the presence of oxygen and converted to energy in the form of ATP. Mitochondria have an inner and outer membrane. The inner membrane has many twists and folds (called cristae), which increase the surface area available to proteins and their associative reactions. The inner membrane encloses a liquid containing DNA, RNA, small ribosomes, and solutes. The DNA in mitochondria is genetically distinct from that in the cell nucleus, and mitochondria can manufacture some of their own proteins independent of the rest of the cell. Each cell can contain thousands of mitochondria, which move about producing ATP in response to the cell's need for chemical energy. It is thought that mitochondria originated as separate, single-celled organisms that became so symbiotic with their hosts as to be indispensable. Mitochondrial DNA is thus considered a remnant of a past existence as a separate organism.

Myocardium – the muscular substance of the heart.

MSG (monosodium **glutamate)** – A white odorless crystalline compound that is a salt of glutamic acid; it is used as a flavor enhancer in foods, an application that may cause Chinese restaurant syndrome in sensitive people, and used intravenously as an adjunct in treating encephalopathies associated with liver disease.

P

Pacemaker – An electronic device implanted beneath the skin for providing a normal heartbeat by electrical stimulation of the heart muscle, used in certain heart conditions.

Perfusionist – a medical technician responsible for blood transfusion and the heart-lung machine during cardiopulmonary surgery.

Physical therapist – the health professional that provides the treatment or management of physical disability, malfunction, or pain by exercise, massage, hydrotherapy, etc., without the use of medicines, surgery, or radiation.

Psychologist – A person trained and educated to perform psychological research, testing, and therapy.

Pulmonary disease – any disease or disorder where lung function is impaired.

Pulmonary specialists – A pulmonary specialist is a medical doctor who has received specialized training and education for the treatment of people who suffer from problems of the lungs.

R

Renal failure – inability of the kidneys to excrete wastes and to help maintain the electrolyte balance

S

Spirometer – an instrument for determining the capacity of the lungs.

Stenosis – a narrowing or stricture of a passage or vessel

Sternum – a compound ventral bone or cartilage that lies in the median central part of the body of most vertebrates above fishes and that in humans is about seven inches (18centimeters) long, consists in the adult of three parts, and connects with the clavicles and the cartilages of the upper seven pairs of ribs called also *breastbone*.

Stent – A slender thread, rod, or catheter inserted into a tubular structure, such as a blood vessel, to provide support during or after anastomosis.

T

Thoracentesis – insertion of a hollow needle or similar instrument into the pleural cavity of the chest in order to drain pleural fluid.

Tranquilizer – One that serves to tranquilize, as soothing music or any of various drugs used to reduce tension or anxiety; an anti-anxiety agent. Any of various drugs used to treat psychotic states; an antipsychotic drug.

U

Urinary catheter – any tube system placed in the body to drain and collect urine from the bladder

USDA – United States Department of Agriculture.

V

Ventilator – A device that circulates fresh air and expels stale or foul air. *Medicine* A respirator.

Vitals – The vital body organs. The parts essential to continued functioning, as of a system. The testing and measurement of those parts.

W

Warfarin – a crystalline anticoagulant coumarin derivative $C_{19}H_{16}O_4$ related to dicumarol that inhibits the production of prothrombin by vitamin K and is used as a rodent poison and in medicine; *also*: its sodium salt $C_{19}H_{15}NaO_4$ used especially in the prevention or treatment of thromboembolic disease

∞

Index

Made in the USA
Middletown, DE
05 August 2018